a LANGE medical book

Vander's Renal Physiology

Ninth Edition

Douglas C. Eaton, PhD
Distinguished Professor of Physiology
and Professor of Pediatrics
Emory University School of Medicine
Atlanta, Georgia

John P. Pooler, PhD
Associate Professor of Physiology
Emory University School of Medicine
Atlanta, Georgia

Mc
Graw
Hill
Education

New York   Chicago   San Francisco   Athens   London   Madrid   Mexico City
Milan   New Delhi   Singapore   Sydney   Toronto

ISBN 978-1-260-01937-7
MHID 1-260-01937-3
ISSN 1548-338X

Notice

Medicine is an ever-changing science. As new research and clinical experience broaden our knowledge, changes in treatment and drug therapy are required. The authors and the publisher of this work have checked with sources believed to be reliable in their efforts to provide information that is complete and generally in accord with the standards accepted at the time of publication. However, in view of the possibility of human error or changes in medical sciences, neither the authors nor the publisher nor any other party who has been involved in the preparation or publication of this work warrants that the information contained herein is in every respect accurate or complete, and they disclaim all responsibility for any errors or omissions or for the results obtained from use of the information contained in this work. Readers are encouraged to confirm the information contained herein with other sources. For example and in particular, readers are advised to check the product information sheet included in the package of each drug they plan to administer to be certain that the information contained in this work is accurate and that changes have not been made in the recommended dose or in the contraindications for administration. This recommendation is of particular importance in connection with new or infrequently used drugs.

This book was set in Adobe Garamond Pro by MPS Limited.
The editors were Michael Weitz and Christina M. Thomas.
The production supervisor was Catherine H. Saggese.
Project management was provided by Anubhav Siddhu of MPS Limited.

This book is printed on acid-free paper.

McGraw-Hill books are available at special quantity discounts to use as premiums and sales promotions, or for use in corporate training programs. To contact a representative please visit the Contact Us pages at www.mhprofessional.com.

To all our students

Contents

Preface

In this newest edition of *Vander's Renal Physiology*, named for Arthur Vander who authored the first five editions many years ago, we approached the task with the same aims as set out in the most recent editions. Those aims are to describe the remarkable workings of the kidneys through carefully worded text and schematic diagrams, using language and concepts that help the reader gain an intuitive grasp of the content. The text stresses two things: the goals of renal processes, to provide context for a given renal activity, and the logic behind renal processes, with attention given to aspects that experience tells us are sticking points for students. As a result the text includes considerable background material that goes beyond strictly renal mechanisms. As any reader of the literature soon discovers, much kidney research today delves deeper and deeper into the intracellular signaling pathways that control renal actions. While this literature is fascinating to read, it is often difficult to place detailed signaling events in the context of overall renal function. Therefore we have focused our coverage on the processes that these intracellular signaling pathways control, while limiting coverage of signaling pathways per se. We revised all sections of the text to bring them up to date. We reworded explanations to make them as logical and clear as possible. This includes replacing or revising several figures. We have provided several aids to help the reader. Each chapter includes a list of key concepts with indicators in the text where those concepts are presented. There are boxed statements scattered throughout the text to help emphasize major points. And there are study questions at the end of each chapter, with an answer key and explanations of the answers at the end of the book.

Renal Functions, Basic Processes, and Anatomy

1

OBJECTIVES

▶ State seven major functions of the kidneys.

▶ Define the balance concept and give examples.

▶ Define the gross structures and their interrelationships: renal pelvis, calyces, renal pyramids, renal medulla (inner and outer zones), renal cortex, papilla.

▶ Define the components of the nephron-collecting duct system and their interrelationships: renal corpuscle, glomerulus, tubule, and collecting-duct system.

▶ Draw the relationship between glomerulus, Bowman's capsule, and the proximal tubule.

▶ Define juxtaglomerular apparatus and describe its three cell types; state the function of the granular cells.

▶ List the individual tubular segments in order; state the segments that comprise the proximal tubule, Henle's loop, and the distal nephron including the collecting-duct system; define principal cells and intercalated cells.

▶ Define the basic renal processes: glomerular filtration, tubular reabsorption, tubular secretion, and tubular production.

▶ Define renal metabolism of a substance and give examples.

RENAL FUNCTIONS

The kidneys are fascinating biological machines. They are multifunction organs that carry out essential tasks far beyond the well-known excretion of waste. Among the most important of these tasks are preservation of blood volume, total body salt and water composition, maintenance of acid-base balance, and assuring bone integrity. The kidneys work cooperatively and interactively with many other organ systems to maintain body function using a coordinated array of cellular mechanisms. This chapter provides a brief account of renal functions and an overview of how the kidneys perform these functions, plus a description of essential renal anatomy. Subsequent chapters delve into the specific renal mechanisms that mediate these functions and how the kidneys interact with other organ systems.

Function 1: Regulation of Water and Electrolyte Balance

 Water, salt, and other electrolytes enter our bodies at variable rates, which perturb the amount and concentration of these substances in the body. The kidneys vary their excretion of electrolytes and water to preserve appropriate levels in the body. In doing so they maintain *balance*, that is, match output to input so as to keep a constant amount in the body. We should think of the body as an open system in steady state. In a steady state there are no net changes (of anything) inside the body. Therefore, ***intake* must equal *output*.** As an example, consider water in the body. Our input of water is sporadic and often not driven in response to body needs. We drink water when thirsty, but we also drink water because it is a component of beverages that we consume for reasons other than hydration. In addition, solid food often contains large amounts of water. The kidneys respond to increases in water content by increasing the output of water in the urine, thereby restoring body water to normal levels. The same principles apply to many electrolytes and other substances that have variable inputs.

We have discussed the importance of balance for water and electrolytes, but another major aspect of water and electrolyte balance is the regulation of plasma osmolality, that is, the summed concentration of dissolved solutes. Osmolality is altered whenever the inputs and outputs of water and dissolved solutes change disproportionately, as when drinking pure water or eating a salty meal. Not only must the kidneys excrete water and solutes to match inputs, they must do so at rates that keep the *ratio* of solutes and water at a nearly constant value (near 290 mOsm/kg).

Of course, renal responses are not instantaneous. Transient changes in the amount of substances in the body are sensed by the kidneys or other organs and activate signaling pathways that lead to changes in renal output.

Besides excreting excess amounts of various substances, the kidneys respond to deficits. While the kidneys cannot generate lost water or electrolytes, they can reduce output to a minimum, thus preserving body stores. One of the major feats of the kidneys is their ability to regulate all of the various electrolytes, total body water, and plasma osmolarity independently. Within limits, we can be on a high-sodium, low-potassium diet or low-sodium, high-potassium diet, with varying water intake and the kidneys adjust excretion of each of these substances to maintain balance. However, the reader should also be aware that being in balance for a substance does not by itself imply a normal state or good health. A person may have an excess or deficit of a substance, yet still be in balance so long as output matches input. This is often the case in chronic disorders of renal function or metabolism.

Function 2: Regulation of Systemic Blood Pressure and Extracellular Fluid Volume

The kidneys work in partnership with cardiovascular system, each one performing a service for the other. In this context, we should remember that cardiac output = heart rate × stroke volume and systemic blood pressure = cardiac output × vascular resistance. The kidney regulates systemic blood pressure in two major ways: (1) determining blood volume which controls cardiac output; and (2) the kidney makes hormones that regulate vascular resistance.

By far the most important task of the kidneys in this regard is to maintain extracellular fluid volume, of which blood plasma is a significant component. This ensures that the vascular space is filled with sufficient volume so that blood can circulate normally. Maintenance of extracellular fluid volume is a result of water and salt balance described above.

In addition to their major role in ensuring adequate volume for the cardiovascular system, the kidneys also participate in the production of vasoactive substances (via the renin-angiotensin-aldosterone system described later) that exert major control over vascular smooth muscle. In turn this influences peripheral vascular resistance and therefore systemic arterial blood pressure. Pathology in this aspect of renal function leads to hypertension.

Function 3: Excretion of Metabolic Waste and Foreign Substances

Our bodies continuously form the end products of metabolic processes. In most cases, those end products are of no use to the body and must be excreted at the same rate as they are produced. These products include urea (from protein), uric acid (from nucleic acids), creatinine (from muscle creatine), urobilin (an end product of hemoglobin breakdown that gives urine much of its color), and the metabolites of various hormones. There are many others, numbering more than 100, including some originating from GI tract bacterial metabolism, all of which must be excreted. These solutes collectively are called uremic retention solutes, or uremic toxins. If the kidneys fail to excrete them and plasma levels rise, there are deleterious effects in the body, a condition called *uremia*. In addition, foreign substances, including many common drugs, are excreted by the kidneys. In many cases the kidneys work in partnership with the liver in the excretion task. The liver metabolizes many organic molecules into water-soluble forms that are more easily handled by the kidneys.

Function 4: Regulation of Red Blood Cell Production

Red blood cell production by the bone marrow is stimulated by the peptide hormone *erythropoietin*. During embryological development erythropoietin is produced by the liver, but in the adult its major source is the kidneys. The renal cells that secrete it are a particular group of interstitial cells in the cortical interstitium near the border between the renal cortex and medulla (see later). The stimulus for its secretion is a reduction in the partial pressure of oxygen in the local environment of the secreting cells. Although renal blood flow is large, renal metabolism is also large, and local oxygenation drops in cases of anemia, blood loss, arterial hypoxia, or inadequate renal blood flow. These conditions all stimulate secretion of erythropoietin. However, in chronic renal failure, renal metabolism falls, resulting in lower oxygen consumption and therefore higher local tissue oxygenation.

This "fools" the erythropoietin-secreting cells into diminished erythropoietin secretion. The ensuing decrease in bone marrow activity is one important causal factor of anemia associated with chronic renal disease.

Function 5: Regulation of Acid-Base Balance

Acids and bases enter the body fluids via ingestion and from metabolic processes. The body must excrete acids and bases to maintain balance and it also has to regulate the concentration of free hydrogen ions (pH) within a limited range. The kidneys accomplish both tasks by a combination of elimination and synthesis. These interrelated tasks are important aspects of renal function and will be explored thoroughly in Chapter 9.

Function 6: Regulation of Vitamin D Production and Regulation of Calcium and Phosphate Balance

Most of the calcium and phosphate in the body is in bone. The kidneys and the GI tract are the major effector sites for calcium and phosphate balance. Both substances are regulated by the interplay between multiple signaling pathways that serve both to preserve bone integrity and to maintain appropriate plasma concentrations. One of these crucial signaling pathways that determine GI absorption of calcium involves vitamin D. While we often think of vitamin D in terms of sunlight or additives to milk, the *active* form of vitamin D (1,25-dihydroxyvitamin D) called calcitriol is produced in the kidneys by conversion of inactive forms of vitamin D. Its rate of synthesis is regulated by hormones that control calcium and phosphate balance and will be discussed in detail in Chapter 10.

Function 7: Gluconeogenesis

Our central nervous system is an obligate user of blood glucose regardless of whether we have just eaten sugary doughnuts or gone without food for a week. Whenever the intake of carbohydrate is stopped for much more than half a day, our body begins to synthesize new glucose (the process of *gluconeogenesis*) from non-carbohydrate sources (amino acids from protein and glycerol from triglycerides). Most gluconeogenesis occurs in the liver, but a substantial fraction occurs in the kidneys, particularly during a prolonged fast.

OVERVIEW OF RENAL PROCESSES

Most of what the kidneys actually do is conceptually speaking fairly straightforward. Of the considerable volume of plasma entering the kidneys each minute from the renal arteries, they transfer (by filtration) about one-fifth of it, minus the larger plasma proteins, into the renal tubules. The volume filtered is huge—typically 180 L per day in a healthy young adult male. They then selectively reabsorb varying fractions of the filtered substances back into the blood, leaving the unreabsorbed portions to be excreted. In some cases, additional amounts are added to the excreted content by secretion or synthesis. There is a division of labor between different regions of the tubules for carrying out these tasks that depends on the type of cell expressed in different regions. In essence, the renal tubules operate like assembly lines; they accept the fluid coming into them, perform some region-specific modification of the fluid, and send it on to the next segment. The final product (urine) contains amounts of each substance necessary to maintain balance for each of the substances.

ANATOMY OF THE KIDNEYS AND URINARY SYSTEM

The operation of the kidneys is intimately connected to their structure. An understanding of renal function requires a grasp of the key aspects of both macroscopic and microscopic structure. The kidneys are bean-shaped organs about the size of a fist. They are located just under the rib cage behind the peritoneal cavity close to the posterior abdominal wall, one on each side of the vertebral column (Figure 1–1). The rounded, outer convex surface of each kidney faces the side of the body, and the indented surface, called the *hilum*, faces the spine. Each hilum is penetrated by blood vessels, nerves, and a ureter. The ureters bend down and travel approximately 30 cm to the bladder. Each ureter within a kidney is formed from several funnel-like structures called major *calyces*,

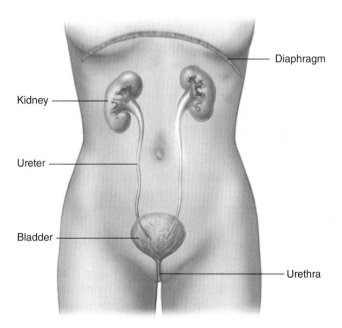

Figure 1–1. Urinary system in a female, indicating the location of the kidneys below the diaphragm and well-above the bladder, which is connected to the kidneys via the ureters. (Reproduced with permission from Widmaier EP, Raff H, Strang KT. *Vander's Human Physiology.* 11th ed. New York: McGraw-Hill; 2008.)

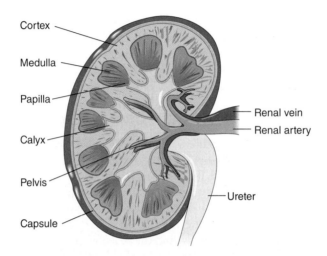

Figure 1–2. Major structural components of the kidney. (Reproduced with permission from Kibble J, Halsey CR. *The Big Picture: Medical Physiology.* New York: McGraw-Hill; 2009.)

which are themselves formed from minor calyces. The minor calyces fit over underlying cone-shaped renal tissue called *pyramids* (Figure 1–2). The tip of each pyramid is called a *papilla* and projects into a minor calyx. The calyces act as collecting cups for the urine formed by the renal tissue in the pyramids. The pyramids are arranged radially around the hilum, with the papillae pointing toward the hilum and the broad bases of the pyramids facing the convex surface of the kidney.

Macroscopically we divide the kidney into cortex and medulla. The pyramids collectively constitute the *medulla* of the kidney. Three dimensionally they are shaped somewhat like acorns, with the tips of the acorns pointed toward the hilum. The *cortex* overlies the tops and sides of the pyramids something like the caps of the acorns. Covering the cortical tissue on the very external surface of the kidney is a thin connective tissue capsule (Figure 1–2).

The working tissue mass of both the cortex and medulla is constructed almost entirely of tubules (nephrons and collecting tubules) and blood vessels (capillaries and capillary-like vessels). Between the tubules and blood vessels is the *interstitium*, which comprises less than 10% of the renal volume. It contains a small amount of interstitial fluid and scattered interstitial cells (fibroblasts and immune cells) that synthesize an extracellular matrix of collagen, proteoglycans, glycoproteins, and several cytokines. And as mentioned, some of these cells synthesize erythropoietin. The kidneys also have a lymphatic drainage system, the function of which is to remove soluble proteins from the interstitium that are too large to penetrate the endothelium of tissue capillaries.

Cortical and medullary tissues differ from each other both structurally and functionally. In the cortex, the tubules and blood vessels are intertwined randomly, something like a plateful of spaghetti. In the medulla, with the exception of some vascular capillaries, the tubules and blood vessels are organized in

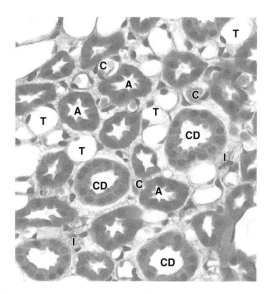

Figure 1–3. Slice through the renal medulla illustrating the close proximity of the tubular and vascular elements. Thin descending limbs (T), thick ascending limbs (A), collecting ducts (CD), and parallel vasa recta (C) are embedded in the interstitium (I) that contains sparse interstitial cells. (Reproduced with permission from Mescher AL. *Junqueira's Basic Histology: Text and Atlas.* 12th ed. New York: McGraw-Hill; 2010.)

parallel arrays like bundles of pencils. In both cases tubules and blood vessels are very close to each other (notice the tight packing of medullary elements shown in Figure 1–3). In addition, the cortex, but not the medulla, contains scattered spherical structures called renal corpuscles. The arrangements of tubules, blood vessels, and renal corpuscles are crucial for renal function, as we will discuss later.

> *The cortex contains renal corpuscles, coiled blood vessels, and coiled tubules; the medulla contains straight blood vessels and straight tubules.*

In the medulla each pyramid is divisible into an outer and inner zone. The outer zone borders the cortex and the inner zone continues to the papilla. The outer zone is further subdivided into an outer stripe and an inner stripe. All these distinctions reflect the organized arrangement of tubules and blood vessels.

THE TUBULAR SYSTEM

Each kidney contains approximately 1 million *nephrons*, which are the tubules that sequentially modify filtered fluid to form the final urine. One nephron is shown diagrammatically in Figure 1–4. Each nephron begins with a spherical filtering component, called the *renal corpuscle*, followed by a long tubule leading out of the renal corpuscle that continues until it merges with

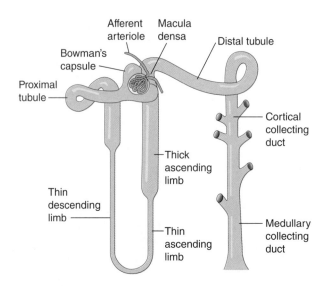

Figure 1–4. Components of the nephron. (Reproduced with permission from Kibble J, Halsey CR: *The Big Picture, Medical Physiology.* New York: McGraw-Hill, 2009.)

the tubules of other nephrons, like a series of tributaries that form a river. The merged tubules are *collecting ducts*, which are themselves long tubes. Collecting ducts eventually merge with other collecting ducts in the renal papilla to form a ureter that conveys urine to the bladder. While nephrons prior to the collecting duct and collecting ducts have different embryological origins, they form a continuous functional unit. For example, the commonly used term "distal nephron" implies elements of both nephrons and the collecting duct.

The Renal Corpuscle

The renal corpuscle is a hollow sphere (*Bowman's capsule*) composed of epithelial cells. It is filled with blood vessels: a compact tuft of interconnected capillary loops called the *glomerulus* (Figure 1–5A). Two closely spaced arterioles penetrate Bowman's capsule at a region called the vascular pole. The afferent arteriole brings blood into the capillaries of the glomerulus and the efferent arteriole drains blood from it. Other cell types—mesangial cells and podocytes—are found in close association with the capillary loops of the glomerulus. Glomerular mesangial cells act as phagocytes and remove trapped material from the basement membrane of the capillaries, while podocytes act as support structures and play an important sieving role in glomerular filtration. The space within Bowman's capsule that is not occupied by capillaries and other cells is called the urinary space or Bowman's space, and it is into this space that fluid filters from the glomerular capillaries before flowing into the first portion of the tubule, located opposite the vascular pole.

The structure and properties of the filtration barrier that separates plasma in the glomerular capillaries from fluid in urinary space are crucial for renal function

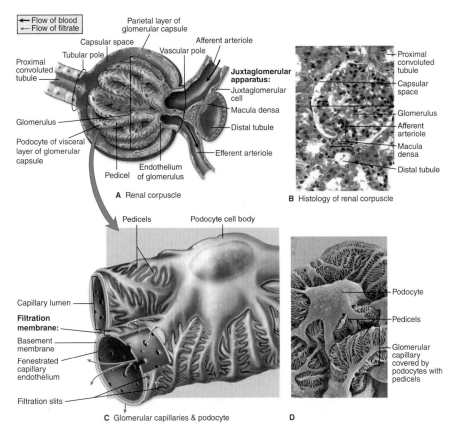

Figure 1–5. **A,** Anatomy of the glomerulus. **B,** Histology of renal corpuscle. **C,** Drawing of podocyte and glomerular capillary. **D,** Scanning EM of podocyte covering glomerular capillaries. (Reproduced with permission from McKinley M, O'Loughlin VD. *Human Anatomy*, 2nd ed. New York: McGraw-Hill; 2008.)

and will be described thoroughly in the next chapter. For now, we note simply that the functional significance of the filtration barrier is that it permits the filtration of large volumes of fluid from the capillaries into Bowman's space, but restricts filtration of plasma proteins such as albumin.

The Tubule

The tubule begins at and leads out of Bowman's capsule on the side opposite the vascular pole. The tubule has a number of segments divided into subdivisions (see Figure 1–6). To avoid excessive detail we usually group together two or more contiguous tubular segments when discussing function. Table 1–1 lists the names and sequence of the various tubular segments. Throughout its length the tubule is made up of a single layer of epithelial cells resting on a basement membrane. The epithelial cells are connected by tight

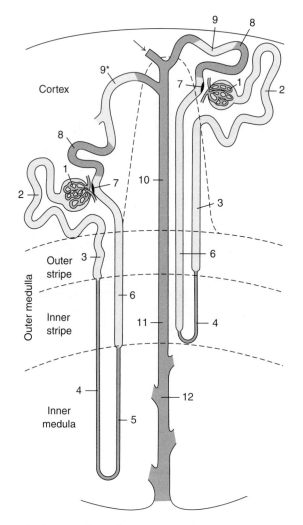

Figure 1–6. Standard nomenclature for structures of the kidney (1988 Commission of the International Union of Physiological Sciences). Shown are a short-looped (right side) and a long-looped, or juxtamedullary nephron (left side), together with the collecting system (not drawn to scale). A cortical medullary ray—the part of the cortex that contains the straight proximal tubules, cortical thick ascending limbs, and cortical collecting ducts— is delineated by a dashed line. 1, renal corpuscle (Bowman's capsule and the glomerulus); 2, proximal convoluted tubule; 3, proximal straight tubule; 4, descending thin limb; 5, ascending thin limb; 6, thick ascending limb; 7, macula densa (located within the final portion of the thick ascending limb); 8, distal convoluted tubule; 9, connecting tubule; 9*, connecting tubule of a juxtamedullary nephron that arches upward to form a so-called arcade (there are only a few of these in the human kidney); 10, cortical collecting duct; 11, outer medullary collecting duct; 12, inner medullary collecting duct. (Reproduced with permission from Kriz W, Bankir L: A standard nomenclature for structures of the kidney. The Renal Commission of the International Union of Physiological Sciences (IUPS), *Am J Physiol.* 1988 Jan;254(1 Pt 2):F1-F8.)

Table 1–1. Terminology for tubular segments

Segments	Collective terms used in text
Proximal convoluted tubule Proximal straight tubule	Proximal tubule
Descending thin limb of the loop of Henle Ascending thin limb of the loop of Henle Thick ascending limb of the loop of Henle	Loop of Henle
Distal convoluted tubule	Distal tubule
Distal tubule Connecting tubule Cortical collecting duct	Distal nephron
Outer medullary collecting duct Inner medullary collecting duct	Medullary collecting duct

> *The renal tubules operate like assembly lines; they accept the fluid coming into them, perform some segment-specific modification of the fluid and send it on to the next segment.*

junctions that physically link the cells together (like the plastic form that holds a six-pack of soft drinks together).

The proximal tubule is the first segment. It drains Bowman's capsule and consists of a coiled segment—the proximal convoluted tubule (sometimes further divided into S1 and S2 segments)—followed by a shorter straight segment—the proximal straight tubule (sometimes called the S3 segment). The coiled segment is entirely within the cortex, while the straight segment descends a short way into the outer medulla (labeled 3 in Figure 1–6). However, most of the length and functions of the proximal tubule are in the cortex.

The next segment is the descending thin limb of the loop of Henle (or simply the descending thin limb). The descending thin limbs of all nephrons begin at the same level, at the point where they connect to straight portions of proximal tubules in the outer medulla. This marks the border between the outer and inner stripe of the outer medulla. While the descending thin limbs of all nephrons begin at the same level, they penetrate down to varying depths in the medulla. At their deepest penetration they abruptly reverse at a hairpin turn and become an ascending portion of the loop of Henle, parallel to the descending portion. In long loops, the ones that have penetrated deepest into the inner medulla, the epithelium of the first portion of the ascending limb remains thin, although different functionally from that of the descending limb. This segment is called the ascending thin limb of Henle's loop, or simply the ascending thin limb (labeled 5 Figure 1–6). Further up the ascending portion the epithelium thickens, and this next segment is called the *thick ascending limb* of Henle's loop, or simply the thick ascending limb. In short loops (depicted in the right side of Figure 1–6) there is no ascending thin portion, and the thick ascending portion begins right at the hairpin loop. All thick ascending limbs begin at the same level, which marks the border between the inner and outer medulla. Therefore, the thick ascending limbs begin at a slightly deeper level in the medulla than do thin descending limbs. Each thick ascending limb rises out of the medulla back into the cortex very close to the same Bowman's capsule from which the tubule originated. Here it passes directly between the afferent and efferent arterioles at the vascular pole of Bowman's capsule. The cells in the thick ascending limb closest to Bowman's capsule (between the afferent and efferent arterioles) are specialized cells known as the macula densa (labeled 7 in Figure 1–6). The macula densa marks the end of the thick ascending limb and the beginning of the distal convoluted tubule (labeled 8 in Figure 1–6). This is followed by the connecting tubule, which leads to the cortical collecting duct, the first portion of which is called the initial collecting tubule.

Connecting tubules from several nephrons merge to form a given *cortical collecting duct* (Figure 1–6). All the cortical collecting ducts then run downward to enter the medulla and become outer medullary collecting ducts, and continue to become inner medullary collecting ducts. These merge to form larger ducts, the last portions of which are called papillary collecting ducts, each of which empties into a calyx of the renal pelvis. Each renal calyx is continuous with the ureter. The tubular fluid, now properly called urine, is not altered after it enters a calyx.

Up to the distal convoluted tubule, the epithelial cells forming the wall of a nephron in any given segment are homogeneous and distinct for that segment. For example, the thick ascending limb contains only thick ascending limb cells. However, beginning in the second half of the distal convoluted tubule the epithelium contains two intermingled cell types. The first constitutes the majority of cells in a particular segment and are usually called *principal cells*. Thus there are segment-specific principal cells in the distal convoluted tubule, connecting tubule, and collecting ducts. Interspersed among the segment-specific cells in these regions are cells of a second type, called *intercalated cells*, that is, they are intercalated between the principal cells. The last portion of the medullary collecting duct contains neither principal cells nor intercalated cells but is composed entirely of a distinct cell type called the inner medullary collecting-duct cells.

> *Loops of Henle penetrate to various depths, then turn upward back to the Bowman's capsules where the tubules began.*

The Juxtaglomerular Apparatus

Earlier we mentioned the macula densa, a portion of the end of the thick ascending limb at the point where this segment comes between the afferent and efferent arterioles at the vascular pole of the renal corpuscle from which the tubule arose. This entire area is known as the juxtaglomerular apparatus (JGA). The JGA, as will be described in Chapter 7, plays an important role in regulating nephron flow and the kidneys' ability to regulate systemic blood pressure. (Do not confuse the term juxtaglomerular *apparatus* with juxtamedullary *nephron*, meaning a nephron with a glomerulus located close to the cortical-medullary border.) Each JG apparatus is made up of three cell types: (1) granular cells, which are differentiated smooth muscle cells in the walls of the afferent arterioles; (2) extraglomerular mesangial cells; and (3) macula densa cells, which are specialized thick ascending limb epithelial cells (see Figure 7–1).

The granular cells are named because they contain secretory vesicles that appear granular in light micrographs. These granules contain the hormone renin (pronounced REE'-nin). As we will describe in Chapter 7, renin is a crucial substance for control of renal function and sodium balance. The extraglomerular mesangial cells are morphologically similar to and continuous with the glomerular mesangial cells, but lie outside Bowman's capsule. The macula densa cells are detectors of the flow rate and composition of the fluid within the nephron at the very end of the thick ascending limb. These detector cells contribute to the control of glomerular filtration rate (GFR—see below) and to the control of renin secretion.

BASIC RENAL PROCESSES

 The working structures of the kidney are the nephrons and collecting tubules into which the nephrons drain. Figure 1–7 illustrates the meaning of several key words that we use to describe how the kidneys function. It is essential that any student of the kidney grasp their meaning.

Filtration is the process by which water and solutes in the blood leave the vascular system through the filtration barrier and enter Bowman's space (a space that is topologically outside the body). *Secretion* is the process of transporting substances into the tubular lumen from the cytosol of epithelial cells that form the walls of the nephron. Secreted substances may originate by synthesis within the epithelial cells or, more often, by leaving the blood and crossing the epithelial layer from the surrounding renal interstitium. *Reabsorption* is the process of moving substances from the lumen across the epithelial layer into the surrounding interstitium and then into the blood.[1] *Excretion* means exit of the substance from the body (i.e., the substance is present in the final urine produced by the kidneys). Synthesis means that a substance is constructed from molecular precursors, and catabolism means the substance is broken down into smaller component molecules. The renal handling of any substance consists of some combination of these processes.

Glomerular Filtration

Urine formation begins with glomerular filtration, the bulk flow of fluid from the glomerular capillaries into Bowman's capsule. The glomerular filtrate (i.e., the fluid

---

[1]We use the term "reabsorption" to describe the movement of filtered substances back into the blood because they are re-entering the blood. "Absorption" describes the original entrance of consumed substances from the GI tract into the blood.

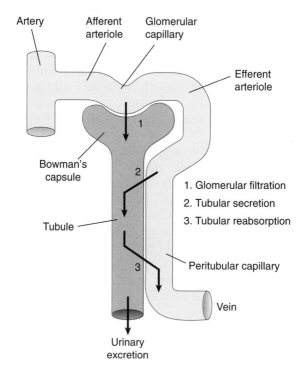

Figure 1–7. Fundamental elements of renal function—glomerular filtration, tubular secretion, and tubular reabsorption—and the association between the tubule and vasculature in the cortex.

within Bowman's capsule) is very much like blood plasma, but contains very little total protein because the large plasma proteins like albumin and the globulins are virtually excluded from moving through the filtration barrier. Smaller proteins, such as many of the peptide hormones, are present in the filtrate, but their mass in total is miniscule compared with the mass of large plasma proteins in the blood. The filtrate contains most inorganic ions and low-molecular-weight organic solutes in virtually the same concentrations as in the plasma. Substances that are present in the filtrate at the same concentration as found in the plasma are said to be freely filtered. (Note that *freely* filtered does not mean *all* filtered. It just means that the amount filtered is in exact proportion to the fraction of plasma volume that is filtered.) Many low-molecular-weight components of blood are freely filtered. Among the most common substances included in the freely filtered category are the ions sodium, potassium, chloride, and bicarbonate; the uncharged organics glucose and urea; amino acids; and peptides like insulin and antidiuretic hormone.

The volume of filtrate formed per unit time is known as the *glomerular filtration rate* (GFR). In a healthy young adult male, the GFR is an incredible 180 L/day (125 mL/min)! Contrast this value with the net filtration of fluid across all the other capillaries in the body: approximately 4 L/day. The implications of this huge

GFR are extremely important. When we recall that the average total volume of plasma in humans is approximately 3 L, it follows that the entire plasma volume is filtered by the kidneys some 60 times a day. The opportunity to filter such huge volumes of plasma enables the kidneys to excrete large quantities of waste products and to regulate the constituents of the internal environment very precisely. One of the general consequences of healthy aging, as well as the effects of many kidney diseases, is a gradual reduction in the GFR (see Chapter 3).

Tubular Reabsorption and Tubular Secretion

The volume and composition of the final urine are quite different from those of the glomerular filtrate. Clearly, almost all the filtered volume must be reabsorbed; otherwise, with a filtration rate of 180 L/day, we would urinate ourselves into dehydration very quickly. As the filtrate flows from Bowman's capsule through the various portions of the tubule, its composition is altered, mostly by removing material (tubular reabsorption) but also by adding material (tubular secretion). As described earlier, the tubule is, at all points, intimately associated with the vasculature, a relationship that permits rapid transfer of materials between the capillary plasma and the lumen of the tubule via the interstitial space.

Most of the tubular transport consists of reabsorption rather than tubular secretion. An idea of the magnitude and importance of tubular reabsorption can be gained from Table 1–2, which summarizes data for a few plasma components that undergo reabsorption. The values in Table 1–2 are typical for a healthy young adult on an average diet. There are at least three important generalizations to be drawn from this table:

1. Because of the huge GFR, the quantities filtered per day are enormous, generally larger than the amounts of the substances in the body. For example, the body of a 70 kg person contains about 42 L of water, but the volume of water filtered each day may be as large as 180 L.
2. Reabsorption of waste products, such as urea, is partial, so that large fractions of their filtered amounts are excreted in the urine.
3. Reabsorption of most "useful" plasma components (e.g., water, electrolytes, and glucose) is either complete (e.g., glucose), or nearly so (e.g., water and most electrolytes), so that very little of the filtered amounts are excreted in the urine.

Table 1–2. Average values for several substances handled by filtration and reabsorption

Substance	Amount filtered per day	Amount excreted	% Reabsorbed
Water, L	180	1.8	99.0
Sodium, g	630	3.2	99.5
Glucose, g	180	0	100
Urea, g	56	28	50

For each plasma substance, a particular combination of filtration, reabsorption, and secretion determines the amount excreted. These processes are subject to physiological control. By triggering changes in the rates of filtration, reabsorption, or secretion when the body content of a substance goes above or below normal, these mechanisms regulate excretion to keep the body in balance. For example, consider what happens when a person drinks a large quantity of water: Within 1 to 2 hours, most of the excess water has been excreted in the urine, mainly as the result of decreased tubular reabsorption. The body is kept in balance for water by increasing excretion.

Metabolism by the Tubules

Although most sources list glomerular filtration, tubular reabsorption, and tubular secretion as the three basic renal processes, we cannot overlook metabolism by the tubular cells. The tubular cells extract organic nutrients from the glomerular filtrate or peritubular capillaries and metabolize them as dictated by the cells' own nutrient requirements. In so doing, the renal cells are behaving no differently than any other cells in the body. In addition, there are other metabolic transformations performed by the kidney that are directed toward altering the composition of the urine and plasma. The most important of these are gluconeogenesis, and the synthesis of ammonium from glutamine and the production of bicarbonate, both described in Chapter 9.

Regulation of Renal Function

Maintaining balance requires *regulation* of renal processes. The mechanisms, to the extent known, will be presented in later chapters. Neural signals, hormonal signals, and intrarenal chemical messengers combine to regulate the processes described above in a manner to allow the kidneys to meet the needs of the body. Neural signals originate in the sympathetic celiac plexus. These sympathetic neural signals exert major control over renal blood flow, glomerular filtration, and the release of vasoactive substances that affect both the kidneys and the peripheral vasculature. Known hormonal signals originate in the adrenal gland, pituitary gland, parathyroid glands, and heart. The adrenal cortex secretes the steroid hormones aldosterone and cortisol, and the adrenal medulla secretes the catecholamines epinephrine and norepinephrine. All of these hormones, but mainly aldosterone, are regulators of sodium and potassium excretion by the kidneys. The posterior pituitary gland secretes the hormone arginine vasopressin (AVP, also called ADH). ADH is a major regulator of water and urea excretion, as well as a contributor to the regulation of sodium excretion. The heart secretes hormones—*natriuretic peptides*—that increase sodium excretion by the kidneys. Besides extrarenal hormones, *intrarenal* chemical messengers (i.e., messengers that originate in one part of the kidney and act in another part, e.g., nitric oxide, puringeric agonists, superoxide, eicosanoids) influence basic renal processes. The advent of genetically modified animals in which these messengers are modified have helped to define the precise roles of these substances.

Two points about regulation should be kept in mind. First, excretion of major substances is regulated by overlapping, redundant controls. Failure of one may be compensated by the operation of another. Second, control systems adapt to chronic conditions and may change in effectiveness over time.

In ensuing chapters of this book we discuss specific mechanisms of reabsorption and secretion. When describing regulation of these mechanisms we are also implying regulation of excretion because any substance present in the tubule and not reabsorbed is destined to be excreted.

Overview of Regional Function

We conclude this chapter with a broad overview of the tasks performed by the individual nephron segments. Later, we examine renal function substance by substance and see how tasks performed in the various regions combine to produce an overall result that is useful for the body.

The glomerulus is the site of filtration—about 150 to 180 L/day for young, healthy females or males. The glomerulus is where the greatest mass of excreted substances enters the nephron. The proximal tubule (convoluted and straight portions together) reabsorbs about two-thirds of the filtered water, sodium, and chloride. It reabsorbs all of the useful organic molecules that the body conserves (e.g., glucose, amino acids). It reabsorbs significant fractions, but by no means all, of many important ions, such as potassium, phosphate, calcium, and bicarbonate. It is the site of secretion of a number of organic substances that are either metabolic waste products (e.g., uric acid, creatinine) or drugs (e.g., penicillin) that clinicians must administer appropriately to make up for renal excretion.

The loop of Henle contains different segments that perform different functions, but the key functions occur in the thick ascending limb. As a whole, the loop of Henle reabsorbs about 20% of the filtered sodium and chloride and 10% of the filtered water. A crucial consequence of these different proportions is that, by reabsorbing relatively more salt than water, the luminal fluid becomes *diluted* relative to normal plasma and the surrounding interstitium. During periods when the kidneys excrete dilute final urine, the role of the loop of Henle in diluting the luminal fluid is crucial.

The end of the loop of Henle contains cells of the *macula densa*, which sense the sodium and chloride content of the lumen and generate signals that influence other aspects of renal function, specifically the *renin-angiotensin system* (discussed in Chapter 7). The distal tubule and connecting tubule together reabsorb some additional salt and water, perhaps 5% of each. The cortical collecting duct is where several connecting tubules join to form a single tubule. Cells of the connecting tubule and cortical collecting duct are strongly responsive to and are regulated by the hormones ADH, angiotensin II, and aldosterone. The latter two hormones enhance sodium reabsorption, while ADH enhances water reabsorption in the collecting ducts. The degree to which these processes are stimulated or not stimulated plays a major role in regulating the amount of solutes and water present in the final urine.

Table 1–3. Normal plasma concentrations of key solutes handled by the kidneys

Sodium	140 ± 5 mEq/L
Potassium	4.1 ± 0.8 mEq/L
Calcium (free fraction)	1.0 ± 0.1 mmol/L
Magnesium	0.9 ± 0.1 mmol/L
Chloride	105 ± 6 mEq/L
Bicarbonate	25 ± 5 mEq/L
Phosphate	1.1 ± 0.1 mmol/L
Glucose	5 ± 1 mmol/L
Urea	5 ± 1 mmol/L
Creatinine	1 ± 0.2 mg/dL
Protein (total)	7 ± 1 g/L

The medullary collecting duct continues the functions of the cortical collecting duct in salt and water reabsorption. In addition, it plays a major role in the excretion of acids and bases. The inner medullary collecting is important in regulating urea excretion. The final result of these various transport processes to keep the various plasma solutes close to the typical values is shown in Table 1–3.

KEY CONCEPTS

1 In addition to excreting waste, the kidneys perform many necessary functions in partnership with other body organ systems.

2 The kidneys regulate the excretion of many substances at a rate that balances their input, thereby maintaining appropriate body content of those substances.

3 A major function of the kidneys is to regulate the volume and osmolality of extracellular fluid volume.

4 The kidneys are composed mainly of tubules and closely associated blood vessels.

5 Each functional renal unit is composed of a filtering component (glomerulus) and a transporting tubular component (the nephron and collecting duct).

6 The tubules are made up of multiple segments with distinct functions.

Basic renal mechanisms consist of filtering a large volume, reabsorbing most of it, and adding substances by secretion, and, in some cases, synthesis.

STUDY QUESTIONS

1–1. Renal corpuscles are located
   a. along the cortico-medullary border.
   b. throughout the cortex.
   c. throughout the cortex and outer medulla.
   d. throughout the whole kidney.

1–2. Relative to the number of glomeruli, how many loops of Henle, and how many collecting ducts are there?
   a. Same number of loops of Henle; same number of collecting ducts.
   b. Fewer loops of Henle; fewer collecting ducts.
   c. Same number of loops of Henle; fewer collecting ducts.
   d. Same number of loops of Henle; more collecting ducts.

1–3. It is possible for the body to be in balance for a substance when
   a. the amount of the substance in the body is constant.
   b. the amount of the substance in the body is higher than normal.
   c. the input of the substance into the body is higher than normal.
   d. in all of these situations.

1–4. The macula densa is a group of cells located in the wall of
   a. Bowman's capsule.
   b. the afferent arteriole.
   c. the end of the thick ascending limb.
   d. the descending thin limb.

1–5. The volume of fluid entering the tubules by glomerular filtration in one day is typically
   a. about three times the renal volume.
   b. about the same as the volume filtered by all the capillaries in the rest of the body.
   c. about equal to the circulating plasma volume.
   d. more than the total volume of water in the body.

1–6. In the context of the kidney, secretion of a substance implies that
   a. it is transported from tubular cells into the tubular lumen.
   b. it is filtered into Bowman's capsule.
   c. it is present in the final urine that is excreted.
   d. it is synthesized by the tubular cells.

Renal Blood Flow and Glomerular Filtration

OBJECTIVES

- ▶ Define renal blood flow, renal plasma flow, glomerular filtration rate, and filtration fraction, and give normal values.
- ▶ State the formula relating flow, pressure, and resistance in any vascular bed.
- ▶ Identify the successive vessels through which blood flows after leaving the renal artery.
- ▶ State the relative resistances of the afferent arterioles and efferent arterioles.
- ▶ Describe how changes in afferent and efferent arteriolar resistances affect renal blood flow.
- ▶ Describe the three layers of the glomerular filtration barrier and define podocyte, foot process, and slit diaphragm.
- ▶ Describe how molecular size and electrical charge determine filterability of plasma solutes; state how protein binding of a low-molecular-weight substance influences its filterability.
- ▶ State the formula for the determinants of glomerular filtration rate, and state, in qualitative terms, why the net filtration pressure is positive.
- ▶ State the reason glomerular filtration rate is so large relative to filtration across other capillaries in the body.
- ▶ Describe how arterial pressure, afferent arteriolar resistance, and efferent arteriolar resistance influence glomerular capillary pressure.
- ▶ Describe how changes in renal plasma flow influence average glomerular capillary oncotic pressure.
- ▶ Define autoregulation of renal blood flow and glomerular filtration rate.

RENAL BLOOD FLOW

The volume of blood flowing through the kidneys is huge relative to their size or metabolic need. Renal blood flow (RBF) is 1 L/min, representing 20% of the resting cardiac output. This is through a tissue that constitutes less than 0.5% of the body mass! Considering that the volume of each kidney is less than 150 cc, this means that each kidney is perfused with over three times its total volume every minute. *All* of this blood is delivered to the cortex. About 5%

to 10% of the cortical blood flow is then directed to the medulla before returning to the general circulation. When discussing RBF it is important to keep in mind the unique arrangement of the renal vasculature. This organization is critical for renal function, over and above the necessity of providing oxygen and nutrients.

Blood enters each kidney at the hilum via a renal artery. After several divisions into smaller arteries blood reaches arcuate arteries that course across the tops of the pyramids between the medulla and cortex. From these, interlobular arteries (also called cortical radial arteries) project upward toward the kidney surface. These arteries give off numerous arterioles, each of which leads to an individual Bowman's capsule and the glomerulus within (see Figure 2–1). These arteries and glomeruli are found *only* in the cortex, never in the medulla. The arterioles leading to glomeruli are called *afferent arterioles* and have important functional characteristics discussed later. In most organs, capillaries recombine to form the beginnings of the venous system, but the glomerular capillaries instead recombine to form another set of arterioles, the *efferent arterioles*. The vast majority of the efferent arterioles soon subdivide into a second set of capillaries called *peritubular capillaries*. These capillaries are widely distributed throughout the cortex in close proximity to the tubular segments. The peritubular capillaries then rejoin to form the veins by which blood ultimately leaves the kidney.

Efferent arterioles of glomeruli situated just above the cortico-medullary border (juxtamedullary glomeruli) do not branch into peritubular capillaries the way most efferent arterioles do. Instead these arterioles descend downward into the outer medulla. Once in the medulla they divide many times to form bundles of parallel vessels called vasa recta (Latin *recta* for "straight" and *vasa* for "vessels"). These bundles of vasa recta penetrate deep into the medulla (see Figure 2–1). Vasa recta on the outside of the vascular bundles give rise to interbundle networks of capillaries that surround Henle's loops and the collecting ducts in the outer medulla. Only the center-most vasa recta supply capillaries in the inner medulla; thus little blood flows into the papilla. The capillaries from the inner medulla re-form into ascending vasa recta that run in close association with the descending vasa recta within the vascular bundles. The structural and functional properties of the vasa recta will be further described in Chapter 6.

The kidneys constitute less than 1% of the body mass but receive 20% of the cardiac output.

Blood flow through the vasa recta into the medulla is far less than cortical blood flow, perhaps 0.1 L/min. Although low relative to cortical blood flow, medullary blood flow is not low in an absolute sense and is quite comparable to blood flow in many other tissues. The significance of the differences between cortical and medullary blood flow and the vascular anatomy is the following: The high blood flow through the peritubular network in the cortex maintains the interstitial environment of the cortical renal tubules very close in composition to that of

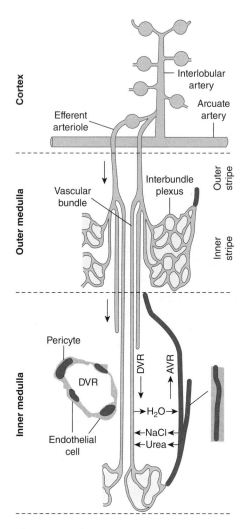

Figure 2–1. The renal microcirculation. Arcuate arteries run just above the cortico-medullary border, parallel to the surface, and give rise to cortical radial (interlobular) arteries radiating toward the surface. Afferent arterioles originate from the cortical radial arteries at an angle that varies with cortical location. Blood is supplied to the peritubular capillaries of the cortex from the efferent flow out of superficial glomeruli. Blood is supplied to the medulla from the efferent flow out of juxtamedullary glomeruli. Efferent arterioles of juxtamedullary glomeruli give rise to bundles of descending vasa recta in the outer stripe of the outer medulla. In the inner stripe of the outer medulla, descending vasa recta and ascending vasa recta returning from the inner medulla run side by side in the vascular bundles, allowing exchange of solutes and water as described in Chapter 6. Descending vasa recta from the bundle periphery supply the interbundle capillary plexus of the inner stripe, whereas those in the center supply blood to the capillaries of the inner medulla. Contractile pericytes in the walls of the descending vasa recta regulate flow. DVR, descending vasa recta. AVR, ascending vasa recta. (Reproduced with permission from Pallone TL, Zhang Z, Rhinehart K: Physiology of the renal medullary microcirculation, *Am J Physiol Renal Physiol.* 2003 Feb;284(2):F253-F266.)

blood plasma throughout the body. In contrast, the lower blood flow and grouping of vascular bundles in the medulla permits an interstitial environment that is quite different from blood plasma. As described in Chapter 6, the interstitial environment in the medulla plays a crucial role in regulating water excretion.

FLOW, RESISTANCE, AND BLOOD PRESSURE IN THE KIDNEYS

 Blood flow in the kidneys obeys the same hemodynamic principles as found in other organs throughout the body. The basic equation for blood flow through any vascular bed is as follows:

$$Q = \frac{\Delta P}{R},$$ Equation 2-1

where Q is blood flow, ΔP is the pressure in the artery supplying the vascular bed minus the pressure in the vein draining it, and R is the total vascular resistance in that vascular bed. The total resistance of a vascular bed is determined by the resistance of individual vessels and their series/parallel connections. The resistance of any single vessel is a function of blood viscosity, vessel length and most of all, vessel radius. As described by Poiseuille's law, the resistance of a cylindrical vessel varies inversely with the fourth power of vessel radius. It takes only a 19% decrease or increase in vessel radius to double or halve vessel resistance. This means that resistance can be controlled physiologically via small changes in vessel radius mediated by arteriolar smooth muscle. Because the kidneys contain so many parallel pathways, that is, glomeruli and associated vessels, total renal vascular resistance is low. In addition, the mean pressure in glomerular capillaries is relatively high compared with peripheral capillaries. The combination of high pressure and low resistance accounts for the high RBF.

The presence of two sets of arterioles (afferent and efferent) and two sets of capillaries (glomerular and peritubular) makes the vasculature of the cortex unusual. The resistances of the afferent and efferent arterioles are about equal under most circumstances and account for most of the total renal vascular resistance. Resistances in arteries preceding afferent arterioles (i.e., cortical radial arteries) and in the capillaries play some role, but we concentrate on the arterioles because these resistances are variable and are the sites of most, if not all, regulation. When the two resistances both change in the same direction (the most common state of affairs), their effects on RBF are additive. When they change in different directions—one resistance increasing and the other decreasing—the changes offset each other and RBF may not change much.

Hydrostatic pressures are much higher in the glomerular capillaries than in the peritubular capillaries. This difference is crucial for function, leading to net filtration in glomerular capillaries and net reabsorption in peritubular capillaries. As blood flows through any vascular resistance the pressure progressively decreases. Pressure at the beginning of a given afferent arteriole is close to mean systemic arterial pressure (~100 mm Hg) and falls to about 60 mm Hg at the point where it

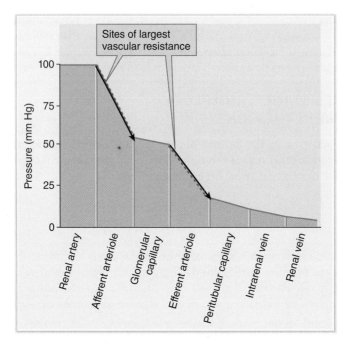

Figure 2–2. Blood pressure decreases as blood flows through the renal vascular network. The largest drops occur in the sites of largest resistance—the afferent and efferent arterioles. The location of the glomerular capillaries, between the sites of high resistance, results in their having a much higher pressure than the peritubular capillaries. (Reproduced with permission from Kibble J, Halsey CR. *The Big Picture: Medical Physiology.* New York: McGraw-Hill; 2009.)

feeds the glomerular capillaries. Because each glomerulus contains so many capillaries in parallel, the effective glomerular resistance is low and pressure remains close to 60 mm Hg during flow through those capillaries. Then pressure decreases again during flow through an efferent arteriole, to about 20 mm Hg at the point where it feeds peritubular capillaries (see Figure 2–2). The high glomerular pressure of about 60 mm Hg is necessary to drive glomerular filtration, whereas the low peritubular capillary pressure of 20 mm Hg is equally necessary to permit the reabsorption of fluid from the renal interstitium.

GLOMERULAR FILTRATION

The glomerular filtrate contains most inorganic ions and low-molecular-weight organic solutes in virtually the same concentrations as in the plasma. It also contains small plasma peptides and a very limited amount of albumin. Filtered fluid must pass through a three-layered glomerular filtration barrier. The first layer, the endothelial cells of the capillaries, is perforated by many large fenestrae ("windows"), like a slice of Swiss cheese, which occupy about 10% of the endothelial surface area. They are freely permeable to everything in the blood except red blood cells and platelets. The middle layer, the capillary basement membrane, is a gel-like acellular meshwork of glycoproteins and proteoglycans, with a structure like a kitchen sponge. The third layer consists of epithelial cells (podocytes) that surround the capillaries and rest on the capillary basement membrane. The podocytes have an unusual octopus-like structure. Arms extend from the soma and wrap around several nearby glomerular capillaries. Small "fingers," called pedicels (or foot processes), extend from each arm and are embedded in the basement membrane (see Figure 1–5C). Pedicels from a given podocyte arm interdigitate with the pedicels from an adjacent podocyte arm. The spaces between the pedicels, called slits, are the passageway through which the glomerular filtrate passes. The pedicels are coated by a thick layer of extracellular material, which partially occludes the slits. Finally, extremely thin processes called slit diaphragms bridge the slits between the pedicels. Slit diaphragms are widened versions of the tight junctions and adhering junctions that link all contiguous epithelial cells together and are like miniature ladders. The pedicels form the sides of the ladder, and the slit diaphragms are the rungs.

Both the slit diaphragms and basement membrane are composed of an array of proteins, and while the basement membrane may contribute to selectivity of the filtration barrier, integrity of the slit diaphragms is essential to prevent excessive leak of plasma protein (albumin). Some protein-wasting diseases are associated with abnormal slit diaphragm structure.

Fixed negative charges in the extracellular matrix of the filtration barrier restrict passage of negatively charged plasma proteins.

The selectivity of the filtration barrier is crucial for renal function. The barrier has to be porous enough to permit free passage of everything that should be filtered, such as water and organic waste, yet restrict plasma proteins that should not be filtered. Selectivity of the barrier is based both on *molecular size* and *electrical charge*. Let us look first at size.

The filtration barrier of the renal corpuscle provides no hindrance to the movement of molecules with molecular weights less than 7000 Daltons (i.e., solutes this small are all freely filtered). This includes all small ions, glucose, urea, amino acids, and many hormones. The filtration barrier almost totally excludes plasma albumin (molecular weight of approximately 66,000 Da). (For simplicity we use molecular weight as the reference for size; in reality, it is molecular radius and shape that is critical.) The hindrance to plasma albumin is not 100%, however, and the glomerular filtrate does contain extremely small quantities of albumin, on the order of 10 mg/L or less. This is only about 0.02% of the concentration of albumin in plasma and is the reason for the use of the phrase "nearly protein-free" earlier. Some small substances are partly or mostly bound to large plasma proteins and are thus not free to be filtered, even though the unbound fractions can easily move through the filtration barrier. This includes hydrophobic hormones of the steroid and thyroid categories and about 40% of the calcium in the blood.

For molecules with a molecular weight ranging from 7000 to 70,000 Da, the amount filtered becomes progressively smaller as the molecule becomes larger (Figure 2–3).

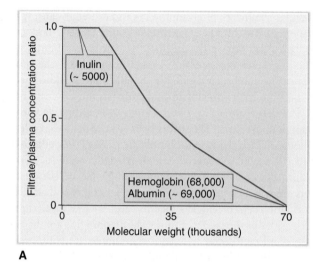

A

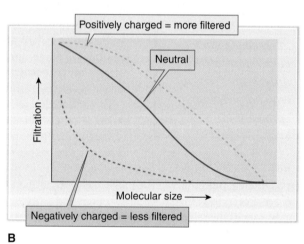

B

Figure 2–3. **A,** As molecular weight (and therefore size) increases, filterability declines, so that proteins with a molecular weight above 70,000 Da are hardly filtered at all. **B,** For any given molecular size, negatively charged molecules are restricted far more than neutral molecules, while positively charged molecules are restricted less. (Reproduced with permission from Kibble J, Halsey CR. *The Big Picture: Medical Physiology.* New York: McGraw-Hill; 2009.)

Thus, many normally occurring small- and medium-sized plasma peptides and proteins are actually filtered to a significant degree. Moreover, when certain small proteins appear in the plasma because of disease (e.g., hemoglobin released from damaged erythrocytes, myoglobin released from damaged muscles, or immunoglobulins in autoimmune diseases like Lupus), considerable filtration of these may occur as well.

 Electrical charge is the second variable determining filterability of macromolecules. For any given size, negatively charged macromolecules are filtered to a lesser extent, and positively charged macromolecules to a greater extent, than neutral molecules. This is because the surfaces of all the components of the filtration barrier (the cell coats of the endothelium, the basement membrane, and the cell coats of the slit diaphragms) contain fixed polyanions, which repel negatively charged macromolecules during filtration. Because almost all plasma proteins bear net negative charge, this electrical repulsion plays a very important restrictive role, enhancing that of purely size hindrance. In other words, if either albumin or the filtration barrier were not charged, even albumin would be filtered to a considerable degree (Figure 2–3). Certain diseases (e.g., Alport's syndrome) that cause glomerular capillaries to become "leaky" to protein do so because negative charges in the membranes are lost.

It must be emphasized that the negative charges in the filtration membranes act as a hindrance only to macromolecules, not to mineral anions or low-molecular-weight organic anions. Thus, chloride and bicarbonate ions, despite their negative charge, are freely filtered.

Direct Determinants of GFR

The value of GFR is a crucial determinant of renal function. It affects the excretion of waste products, and because its normal value is so large, it affects the excretion of all the substances that are handled by downstream tubular elements, particularly salt and water. Regulation of the GFR is straightforward in terms of physical principles, but complex functionally because there are many signals impinging on the controllable elements.

The rate of filtration in the glomeruli is determined by the hydraulic permeability of the capillaries (including in this case, all elements of the filtration barrier), their total surface area, and the net filtration pressure (NFP) acting across them.

Rate of filtration = hydraulic permeability × surface area × NFP   Equation 2-2

Because it is difficult to estimate the surface area of the glomerular capillaries, a parameter called the filtration coefficient (K_f) is used to denote the product of the hydraulic permeability and surface area.

The net filtration pressure is the algebraic sum of the hydrostatic pressures and the osmotic pressures resulting from protein—the oncotic, or colloid osmotic pressures—on the two sides of the capillary wall. There are four pressures to consider: two hydrostatic pressures and two oncotic pressures. These are known as Starling forces. In the glomerular capillaries:

$$\text{NFP} = (P_{GC} - P_{BC}) - (\pi_{GC} - \pi_{BC}),\qquad \text{Equation 2-3}$$

where P_{GC} is glomerular capillary hydrostatic pressure, π_{BC} is oncotic pressure of fluid in Bowman's capsule, P_{BC} is hydrostatic pressure in Bowman's capsule, and π_{GC} is oncotic pressure in glomerular capillary plasma, shown schematically in Figure 2–4, along with typical average values.

Because there is normally little total protein in Bowman's capsule, π_{BC} may be taken as zero. Accordingly, the overall equation for GFR becomes

$$\text{GFR} = K_f \cdot (P_{GC} - P_{BC} - \pi_{GC}).\qquad \text{Equation 2-4}$$

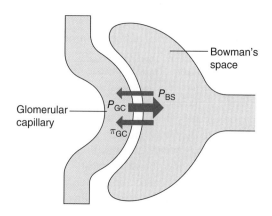

Forces	mmHg
Favoring filtration:	
Glomerular capillary blood pressure (P_{GC})	60
Opposing filtration:	
Fluid pressure in Bowman's space (P_{BS})	15
Osmotic force due to protein in plasma (π_{GC})	29
Net glomerular filtration pressure = $P_{GC} - P_{BS} - \pi_{GC}$	16

Figure 2–4. Forces involved in glomerular filtration as described in the text. (Reproduced with permission from Widmaier EP, Raff H, Strang KT. *Vander's Human Physiology.* 11th ed. New York: McGraw-Hill; 2008.)

Figure 2–5 shows that the hydrostatic pressure is nearly constant within the glomeruli, but the *oncotic* pressure in the glomerular capillaries *does* change substantially along the length of the glomeruli. As water is filtered out of the vascular space it leaves most of the protein behind, thereby increasing protein concentration and, hence, the oncotic pressure of the unfiltered plasma remaining in the glomerular capillaries. Mainly because of this large increase in oncotic pressure, the net filtration pressure decreases from the beginning of the glomerular capillaries to the end.

The net filtration pressure when averaged over the whole length of the glomerulus is about 16 mm Hg (see Figure 2–4). This average net filtration pressure is higher than found in most non-renal capillary beds. Taken together with a very high value for K_f, it accounts for the enormous filtration of 180 L of fluid/day (compared with 3 L/day or so in all other capillary beds combined).

Under resting conditions the GFR is held nearly constant by the process of autoregulation described below. However, it shows a regular diurnal variation, decreases considerably during exercise and is altered in a variety of disease states. To understand control of the GFR, it is essential to see how a change in any one factor affects GFR under the assumption that all other factors are held constant.

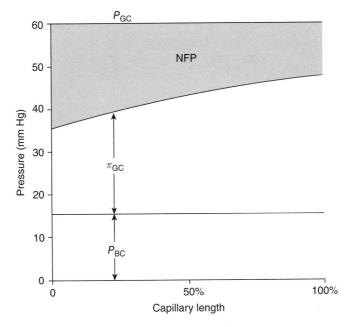

Figure 2–5. Forces affecting glomerular filtration along the length of the glomerular capillaries. Note that the oncotic pressure within the capillaries (π_{GC}) rises due to loss of water and that the net filtration pressure (shaded region) decreases as a result.

Glomerular Capillary Hydrostatic Pressure (P_{GC})

In order to maintain GFR at a given level, the hydrostatic pressure in the glomerular capillaries must remain nearly constant. This pressure is influenced by a number of factors. We can understand the situation using the analogy of a leaky garden hose. If pressure in the pipe feeding the hose rises, the pressure in the hose and, hence, the rate of leak will also rise. But resistances in the hose also affect the leak. If we pinch the hose upstream from the leak, pressure at the region of leak decreases and less water leaks out. However, if we pinch the hose beyond the leak, this *increases* pressure at the region of leak and increases the leak rate. These same principles apply to P_{GC} and GFR. First, a change in renal arterial pressure causes a change in glomerular pressure in the same direction. If resistances remain constant, glomerular pressure rises and falls as renal artery pressure rises and falls. Second, changes in the resistance of the afferent and efferent arterioles have *opposite* effects on glomerular pressure. An increase in afferent arteriolar resistance, which is *upstream* from the glomerulus, is like compressing the hose above the leak—it decreases glomerular pressure. An increase in efferent arteriolar resistance is *downstream* from the glomerulus and is like compressing the hose beyond the leak—it increases glomerular pressure. Of course dilation of the afferent arteriole raises glomerular pressure and hence GFR, while dilation

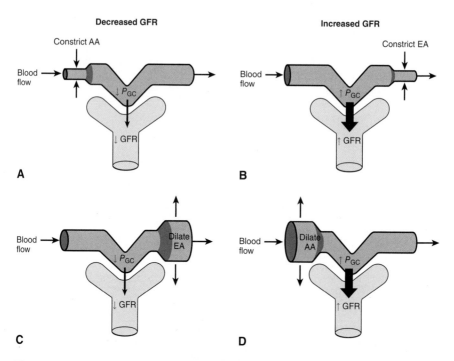

Figure 2–6. Effect of changes in resistance on GFR. Constricting the afferent arteriole (AA) or dilating the efferent arteriole (EA) lead to a decreased GFR, while dilating the AA or constricting the EA lead to increased GFR. (Reproduced with permission from Widmaier EP, Raff H, Strang KT. *Vander's Human Physiology.* 11th ed. New York: McGraw-Hill; 2008.)

of the efferent arteriole lowers glomerular pressure and GFR. It should also be clear that when the afferent and efferent arteriolar resistances both change in the same direction (i.e., they both increase or decrease), they exert opposing effects on glomerular pressure but additive effects on RBF.

What is the significance of this? It means the kidney can regulate glomerular pressure and, hence, GFR *independently* of RBF. The concepts described above are illustrated in Figure 2–6.

Hydrostatic Pressure in Bowman's Capsule (P_{BC})

Changes in pressure within Bowman's space are usually of very minor importance. However, obstruction anywhere along the tubule or in the external portions of the urinary system (e.g., the ureter) increases the tubular pressure everywhere proximal to the occlusion, all the way back to Bowman's capsule. The result is to decrease GFR.

Oncotic Pressure in Glomerular Capillary Plasma (π_{GC})

Oncotic pressure in the plasma at the very beginning of the glomerular capillaries is the oncotic pressure of systemic arterial plasma. Accordingly, a decrease in arterial plasma protein concentration, as occurs, for example, in liver disease, decreases arterial oncotic pressure and tends to increase GFR, whereas increased arterial oncotic pressure tends to reduce GFR.

However, recall that glomerular oncotic pressure is the same as arterial oncotic pressure only at the very beginning of the glomerular capillaries; glomerular oncotic pressure increases somewhat as protein-free fluid filters out of the capillary, concentrating the protein left behind. This means that net filtration pressure and, hence, filtration progressively decrease along the capillary length. Accordingly, anything that causes a steeper increase in glomerular oncotic pressure tends to lower average net filtration pressure and hence GFR.

Such a steep increase in oncotic pressure occurs in conditions of low RBF. When RBF is low, the filtration process removes a relatively larger fraction of the plasma, leaving a smaller volume of plasma behind in the glomeruli still containing all the plasma protein. The glomerular oncotic pressure reaches a final value at the end of the glomerular capillaries that is higher than normal. This lowers average net filtration pressure and, hence, GFR. Conversely, a high RBF, all other factors remaining constant, causes glomerular oncotic pressure to increase less steeply and reach a final value at the end of the capillaries that is less than normal, which increases the GFR.

Since blood is composed of cells and plasma, we can describe the flow of plasma per se, the renal *plasma* flow (RPF). Variations in the relative amounts of plasma that are filtered can be expressed as a *filtration fraction*: the ratio GFR/RPF, which is normally about 20%, that is, about 20% of the plasma entering the kidney is removed from the blood and put into the Bowman's space. The increase in glomerular oncotic pressure along the glomerular capillaries is directly proportional to the filtration fraction (i.e., if relatively more of the plasma is filtered, the increase in glomerular oncotic pressure is greater). If the filtration fraction has changed, it is certain that there has also been a proportional change in glomerular oncotic pressure and that this has played a role in altering GFR.

Filtration Coefficient (K_f)

Changes in K_f are caused most often by glomerular disease, but may occasionally be subject to normal physiological control. The details are still not completely clear, but chemical messengers released within the kidneys cause contraction of podocytes. Such contraction is thought to stabilize the fragile capillaries in the face of changes in renal arterial pressure. It is also possible that this restricts flow through some of the capillary loops, effectively reducing the area available for filtration, K_f, and, hence GFR. It should be noted that the major cause of decreased GFR in normal aging and renal disease is not a change in the filtration coefficient within individual glomeruli, but rather a decrease in the number of functioning nephrons. This reduces whole kidney K_f.

Filtered Load

A term we use in other chapters is filtered load. It is the amount of substance that is filtered per unit time. For freely filtered substances, the filtered load is the product of GFR and plasma concentration. Consider sodium. Its normal plasma concentration is 140 mEq/L, or 0.14 mEq/mL. A normal GFR in healthy young adult males is 125 mL/min, so the filtered load of sodium is 0.14 mEq/mL × 125 mL/min = 17.5 mEq/min. We can do the same calculation for any other substance, being careful in each case to be aware of the unit of measure in which concentration is expressed. The filtered load is what is presented to the rest of the nephron to handle. The filtered load varies with plasma concentration and GFR. An increase in GFR, at constant plasma concentration, increases the filtered load, as does an increase in plasma concentration at constant GFR. Variations in filtered load play a major role in the renal handling of many substances.

AUTOREGULATION

It is important for the kidneys to keep the GFR within a limited range. If GFR is too low for an extended period of time, there will be insufficient excretion of waste substances. Even more important on a short-term basis is the necessity to allow appropriate loads of salt and water to enter the tubule. Most of the time this means keeping GFR relatively constant in the face of factors that change it. We say this recognizing that GFR decreases at night in a regular diurnal rhythm and falls substantially during exercise. In the latter case the body prioritizes perfusion of working muscle over a transient reduction in renal excretion.

The most important of the factors tending to change GFR is renal artery pressure. In the healthy kidney, renal artery pressure is virtually the same as systemic arterial pressure. Arterial pressure is by no means constant, regularly showing peaks and valleys of 20% or more. Its potential effect on GFR is so strong that urinary excretion would tend to vary widely with ordinary daily excursions of arterial pressure. Also, vascular pressure in the thin-walled glomerular capillaries is higher than in capillaries elsewhere in the body and hypertensive damage ensues if this pressure is too high. To protect the glomerular capillaries from hypertensive damage and to preserve a healthy GFR at different arterial pressure values, changes in GFR and RBF are minimized by several mechanisms that we collectively call autoregulation.

Fractional changes in renal artery pressure are *magnified* in terms of fractional changes in net filtration pressure. We can illustrate this via a hypothetical rise in mean arterial pressure from 100 to 120 mm Hg (a 20% increase). Such a modest rise occurs many times throughout the day in association with changes in excitement level and activity. Using values from Table 2–1, glomerular capillary pressure is originally 60 mm Hg and net filtration pressure is 16 mm Hg. If all renal vascular resistances remained constant, glomerular capillary pressure would increase by about half of 20 mm Hg, that is, from 60 to 70 mm Hg. The pressure opposing filtration would not change, so the net filtration pressure would initially increase from 16 to 26 mm Hg, that is, a 62% increase. Without autoregulatory responses, the GFR would more than double. A similar argument applies to decreases in renal artery pressure. This emphasizes why it is so important to maintain glomerular capillary pressure at the right value.

Table 2–1. Estimated forces involved in glomerular filtration in humans

Forces	Afferent end of glomerular capillary (mm Hg)	Efferent end of glomerular capillary (mm Hg)
1. Favoring filtration Glomerular-capillary hydraulic pressure, P_{GC}	60	58
2. Opposing filtration a. Hydraulic pressure in Bowman's capsule, P_{BC}	15	15
b. Oncotic pressure in glomerular capillary, π_{GC}	21	33
3. Net filtration pressure (1−2)	24	10

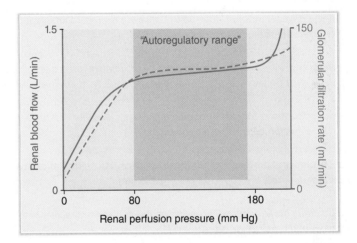

Figure 2–7. Autoregulation of renal blood flow (RBF) and glomerular filtration rate (GFR). Over the span of renal perfusion pressure (pressure in renal artery minus pressure in renal vein) from 80 to about 170 mm Hg, RBF and GFR rise only modestly as renal perfusion pressure increases. Outside of this range, however, the changes are much greater. (Reproduced with permission from Kibble J, Halsey CR. *The Big Picture: Medical Physiology.* New York: McGraw-Hill; 2009.)

Now, what actually happens in the face of changes in mean arterial pressure? As is the case in many organs, blood flow does not change in proportion to changes in arterial pressure. The changes are blunted. A rise in driving pressure is counteracted by a rise in vascular resistance that *almost* offsets the rise in pressure. The word "almost" is crucial here. Higher driving pressures do indeed lead to higher flow but not proportionally. Consider Figure 2–7. Within the range of mean arterial pressures commonly found in the human body (in the region labeled "Autoregulatory range"), GFR and RBF vary only modestly when mean arterial pressure changes. This is partly a result of the myogenic response, which is the contraction or relaxation of arteriolar smooth muscle in response to changes in

> *Autoregulation prevents large changes in GFR in the face of changes in arterial pressure.*

vascular pressures. Autoregulation is also partly the result of intrarenal signals that affect vascular resistance called tubuloglomerular feedback (TG feedback, see Chapter 7). The myogenic response is very fast-acting (within 1 second) and protects the glomeruli from short-term fluctuations in blood pressure, while TG feedback helps maintain an appropriate filtered load of sodium and waste products.

KEY CONCEPTS

 The kidneys have a very large blood flow relative to their mass that is regulated for functional reasons rather than metabolic demand.

 Glomerular capillary pressure is determined by the relative resistances of afferent arterioles, which precede the glomerulus, and efferent arterioles, which follow it.

 Glomerular filtration proceeds through a three-layered barrier that restricts filtration of large macromolecules such as albumin.

 Negative surface charge on the filtration barrier restricts filtration of negatively charged solutes more than positively charged solutes.

 The glomerular filtration rate (GFR) is determined by the permeability of the filtration barrier and net filtration pressure (NFP).

 Net filtration pressure (NFP) varies mainly with hydrostatic and oncotic pressures in the glomerular capillaries.

 Control of the resistances of the afferent and efferent arterioles permits independent control of glomerular filtration rate and renal blood flow.

 Autoregulation of vascular resistances keeps GFR within limits in the face of large variations in arterial pressure.

STUDY QUESTIONS

2–1. Blood enters the renal medulla immediately after passing through which vessels?
   a. Arcuate arteries
   b. Peritubular capillaries
   c. Afferent arterioles
   d. Efferent arterioles

2–2. Which cell type is the main determinant of the filterability of plasma solutes?
   a. Mesangial cell.
   b. Podocyte.
   c. Endothelial cell.
   d. Vascular smooth muscle.

2–3. Which one of the following is NOT subject to physiological control on a moment-to-moment basis?
   a. Hydrostatic pressure in glomerular capillaries.
   b. Selectivity of the filtration barrier.
   c. Filtration coefficient.
   d. Resistance of efferent arterioles.

2–4. A substance is freely filtered and has a certain concentration in peripheral plasma. You would expect the substance to have virtually the same concentration in
   a. the glomerular filtrate.
   b. the afferent arteriole.
   c. the efferent arteriole.
   d. all of these places.

2–5. In the face of a 20% decrease in arterial pressure, GFR decreases by only 2%. What could account for this finding?
   a. The resistances of the afferent and efferent arterioles both decrease equally.
   b. Glomerular mesangial cells contract.
   c. Efferent arteriolar resistance increases.
   d. Afferent arteriolar resistance increases.

2–6. The hydrostatic pressure within the glomerular capillaries
   a. is much higher than in most peripheral capillaries.
   b. is about the same as in the peritubular capillaries.
   c. decreases markedly along the length of the capillaries.
   d. is generally lower than the oncotic pressure in the glomerular capillaries.

Clearance and Measures of Renal Function

THE CLEARANCE CONCEPT

As outlined in Chapter 1, the body constantly removes metabolic waste products, ingested substances, and excess salt and water from the body by a number of means, including disposal in the urine, in the feces, biochemical transformation in the liver, and for volatile substances, exhalation. The rate of removal of any substance can be expressed in several ways, a common one being the plasma half-life, that is, the time it takes for the concentration in the plasma to be reduced by 50%. Another way to express removal rate is clearance, which is the *volume of plasma per unit time from which all of a specific substance is removed.* Clearance in a biomedical context has both a general meaning and a specific renal meaning. The general meaning is simply that a substance is removed from the plasma by any of the mechanisms mentioned above. Its quantitative measure is called the metabolic clearance rate. Renal clearance, on the other hand, means that the substance is removed from the plasma only by the kidneys and is either excreted in the urine or catabolized by the renal tubules.

> *Clearance measures the volume of plasma from which all of a substance is removed in a given time.*

Compare how the body handles two substances with similar-sounding names but very different properties: *inulin* and insulin. Insulin is the familiar pancreatic hormone involved in regulating blood glucose. It is a protein with a molecular weight of 5.8 kDa and is small enough to be freely filtered by the glomerulus. Once in Bowman's space, it moves along with every other filtered substance into the proximal convoluted tubule, where it is largely taken up by endocytosis and degraded into its constituent amino acids. Very little insulin escapes this uptake, and very little of the filtered insulin makes it all the way to the urine. Thus, the kidneys take part in clearing insulin from the blood. However, the body has additional mechanisms for removing insulin from the blood and its metabolic clearance rate is very high (half-life less than 10 minutes). Let us contrast this with inulin. *Inulin* is a polysaccharide starch of about 5-kDa molecular weight that is not usually found in the body. Like insulin, it is freely filtered by the glomerulus, but it is not reabsorbed or secreted by the nephron. All the inulin that is filtered flows through the nephron and appears in the urine. Its plasma half-life is more than an hour. Since the kidneys are the only excretion route, the clearance of inulin specifically indicates *renal* clearance. As we will see, this makes inulin a very special substance for assessing renal function.

The practical utility of measuring the renal clearance of inulin and several other substances described later is to measure GFR. Evaluation of GFR is used clinically as an overall assessment of renal health. Repeated assessments of GFR over a period of time can indicate whether renal function is stable or deteriorating. It is also important to know the GFR when using pharmacological agents that are toxic to the kidneys (e.g., contrast agents, immunosuppressant, or chemotherapeutic drugs), since slow clearance increases the chances of renal damage. In addition, GFR offers some indication of the ability of the kidneys to rid the body of uremic toxins, although many of these enter the tubule via secretion in addition to filtration.

CLEARANCE UNITS

The units of clearance are *volume* per time (*not* amount of a substance per time). The volume is the volume of plasma that has all of the substance removed from it. Equivalently, for substances that are not metabolized by the kidneys, it is the volume that supplied the amount appearing in the urine. The reader should appreciate that removing all of a substance from a small volume of

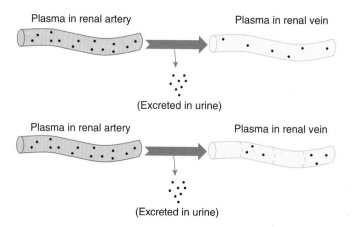

Figure 3–1. Renal clearance. When plasma is cleared of a solute, the solute concentration in venous plasma leaving the kidney is lower than in arterial plasma entering the kidney, as shown in the upper part of the figure. This is equivalent to dividing the plasma into segments in which all the solute is removed from some segments and none from others, as shown in the bottom of the figure. The volume of plasma from which all the solute has been removed, when expressed on a time basis, is the clearance of the solute in units of volume per time.

plasma is the same as removing only some of it from a larger volume, which is actually the way the kidneys do it. If all of substance is removed from a given volume in 1 hour, this is equivalent to removing half of it from twice that volume, or one-quarter of it from four times the volume, etc. The clearance is the same in all these cases.

These concepts are illustrated in Figure 3–1. As the kidneys clear a substance, plasma leaving the kidney in the renal vein has a lower concentration of the substance than does plasma entering the kidney in the renal artery. This can be pictured as dividing the plasma into sequential segments in which all of the substance is removed from some segments (the cleared volumes) and none from others.

Quantification of Clearance

Clearance of any given substance is most easily quantified when its only removal route is excretion in the urine, that is, it is not metabolized. Consider a substance X that is excreted in the urine. The amount of X removed from plasma equals the amount excreted in the urine. The *amount* removed from the plasma in a given time is the product of the volume of plasma cleared per unit time (C_x) and the plasma concentration (P_x) (Equation 3-1). That same amount now appearing in the urine during this time is the product of the urine flow rate (V) and the urine concentration of X (U_x) (Equation 3-2). We equate these quantities in Equation 3-3 and rearrange to solve for clearance in Equation 3-4 expressed in the proper units—*volume* per time.

$$\text{amount cleared/time} = C_x \cdot P_x \qquad \text{Equation 3-1}$$

$$\text{amount in urine/time} = V \cdot U_x \qquad \text{Equation 3-2}$$

$$C_x \cdot P_x = V \cdot U_x \qquad \text{Equation 3-3}$$

$$C_x = V \cdot U_x / P_x \qquad \text{Equation 3-4}$$

While addressing the quantification of clearance, note that the product of urine flow rate and urine concentration of X (Equation 3-2) is excretion rate. Therefore, we can also state that *the clearance of substance X is the excretion rate divided by the plasma concentration.*

As described above, inulin is freely filtered and neither reabsorbed nor secreted. Thus, once filtered, it must flow through the nephron into the urine (Figure 3–2). The volume of plasma cleared of inulin is the volume filtered. Therefore, inulin clearance equals the glomerular filtration rate (GFR). Inulin clearance is indeed the hallmark experimental method of measuring the GFR.

Depending on how they are handled by the kidneys, different substances may have renal clearances that are higher or lower than the GFR. Para-aminohippurate (PAH) is a small (molecular weight of 194 Da) water-soluble organic anion not normally found in the body, which is used experimentally. It is freely filtered and also avidly secreted by the proximal tubule epithelium. Therefore much more is removed than just the amount that is filtered. The secretion rate is saturable. (That is, there is a maximum rate of PAH secretion into the tubule. Such a tubular maximum, or T_m, is common in transport systems; [see Chapter 4]). However, at low plasma concentrations, almost all of the PAH

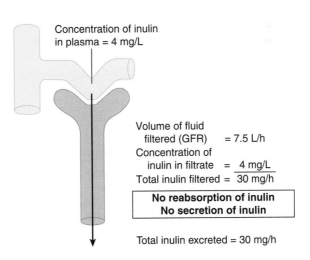

Figure 3–2. Renal handling of inulin. All filtered inulin is excreted. Since the volume of plasma cleared of inulin is the volume filtered, the inulin clearance equals the GFR.

entering the kidney is removed from the plasma and excreted in the urine. Its clearance, therefore, is nearly as great as the renal plasma flow (i.e., much greater than the GFR). In fact, the PAH clearance can be used experimentally as a measure of renal plasma flow, usually called the effective renal plasma flow to indicate that its value is slightly less than the true renal plasma flow.

In general, if we know the GFR and the clearance of a given freely filtered substance, then any difference between its clearance and GFR represents net secretion or reabsorption. If the clearance is greater than the GFR, there must have been net secretion, while a clearance less than the GFR indicates net reabsorption. If the clearance of a substance exactly equals the GFR, then there has been no *net* reabsorption or secretion. The word *net* in this description is important because, as we will see in later chapters, a number of substances are reabsorbed in certain regions of the nephron and secreted in other regions. The net result of these processes is the sum of everything that happens along the nephron. Of course, if a substance is *not* freely filtered, low clearance may simply indicate that little of the substance entered the tubule in the first place.

Practical Methods of Measuring GFR: Clearance of Exogenous Agents and Endogenously Produced Substances

 The most accurate measures of GFR involve administration of exogenous agents. The gold standard for measuring GFR is inulin clearance, and this method is commonly used in research studies. The method is cumbersome, however, because inulin must either be infused at a rate sufficient to keep its plasma concentration constant during the period of urine formation and collection, or there must be multiple samplings and a complex regression analysis. Other measures of renal function that

> *Creatinine clearance is the common method to measure GFR.*

depend upon administration of exogenous agents are occasionally used as alternatives when renal function must be determined with high accuracy to evaluate the progression of chronic kidney disease. All of these agents have in common that they are primarily removed from the body by the kidneys, and are freely filtered, not secreted, and not reabsorbed, that is, they behave like inulin. Many are radioactive to increase sensitivity and ease of measurements (e.g., ^{125}I-iothalamate, ^{59}Cr-EDTA, and ^{99m}Tc-DTPA). These agents produce extremely accurate measurements of GFR and are easier to administer than inulin, but all suffer from having to deal with the handling and disposal of radioactive materials. A newer approach using DTPA (diethylenetriaminepentaacetic acid) bound to gadolinium has promise, but is not yet in common use. All of these agents are invasive and so some less invasive procedure is typically used.

For routine assessment of GFR in patients, there are much easier methods: either direct measurement of creatinine clearance, or more commonly, *estimates* of GFR using plasma levels of creatinine or cystatin C. Creatinine is an end

> *Plasma creatinine/cystatin C concentrations vary inversely with GFR and are a practical indicator of how well the kidneys are filtering.*

product of creatine metabolism and is exported into our blood continuously by skeletal muscle. The rate is proportional to skeletal muscle mass, and to the extent that muscle mass remains constant in an individual, the creatinine production is constant. Creatinine is freely filtered and not reabsorbed. To measure a patient's creatinine clearance, the urine is collected for 24 hours, and a blood sample is taken sometime during the collection period. Blood and urine are assayed for creatinine concentration, and we apply the clearance formula (Equation 3-4) to yield creatinine clearance.

One problem with creatinine is that a small amount is secreted by the proximal tubule. Because of the secretion, creatinine clearance is slightly higher than the GFR, normally by about 10% to 20%. For routine assessment of GFR, this degree of error is acceptable. For a patient with a very low GFR, the secreted component comprises a relatively larger fraction of the total amount excreted; therefore, the creatinine clearance more severely overestimates GFR in patients with a very low GFR than in those with higher GFR values. Nevertheless, because of low cost and convenience, creatinine clearance is a useful method for assessment of patient GFR and the integrity of renal filtration.

Plasma Creatinine and Cystatin C to Estimate GFR

Measuring the clearance of creatinine or any other substance takes time, and it is often necessary to obtain a value for GFR more quickly. Therefore, methods have been developed that require only a single blood sample. These methods require an endogenous substance which is produced at a fixed rate and which is primarily removed from the body via the kidney. In addition, the substance must be freely filtered and minimally secreted or reabsorbed. For such substances, there will be an inverse relation between plasma concentration and GFR (e.g., Figure 3–3).

As discussed above, creatinine is one such substance; another such substance is cystatin C. Cystatin C is a 13.3-kDa polypeptide that is continuously produced at a relatively constant rate in almost all tissues of the body. It is almost completely cleared from the bloodstream by glomerular filtration. Following filtration, it is taken up by proximal tubule cells and degraded into its constituent amino acids. Nonetheless, all of its removal from the blood is via the kidneys. Even though it is not excreted in the urine, all the cystatin C that is filtered is removed from the body (degraded), and thus the same inverse relation between GFR and creatinine is also true for plasma cystatin C.

A healthy person's plasma creatinine concentration is about 1 mg/dL; cystatin C concentration is about 0.07 mg/dL. Both remain stable because the amount removed by the kidneys is equal to the amount produced each day. If the GFR suddenly decreases by 50% because of an obstruction in the renal artery, the

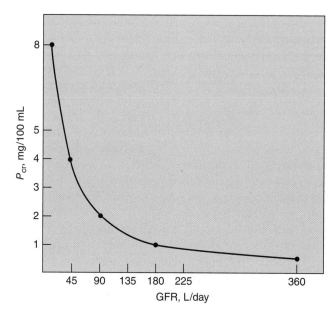

Figure 3–3. Steady-state relation between plasma creatinine and GFR for a person with a normal creatinine production. When GFR is low, plasma creatinine rises to high levels, making plasma creatinine a convenient indicator of GFR.

person filters only 50% as much creatinine (or cystatin C) as normal. Therefore, creatinine excretion is reduced by 50% and the person transiently goes into positive creatinine balance. However, despite the persistent 50% GFR reduction, the plasma creatinine does not continue to rise indefinitely; rather, it stabilizes at 2 mg/dL (i.e., after it has doubled). Half the previous volume is being filtered, but that volume has twice the previous creatinine concentration, so the amount excreted returns to normal. The increase in plasma concentration results directly from the decrease in GFR. Therefore, plasma creatinine gives a reasonable indication of GFR. Of course, cystatin C concentration would behave in a similar fashion and also give an indication of GFR.

Neither plasma creatinine nor plasma cystatin C is completely an accurate indicator of GFR. Creatinine is inaccurate because as mentioned before some creatinine is secreted, and creatinine production may be altered in certain disease states that affect muscle mass or liver function. It may also increase transiently when ingesting large amounts of red meat. Creatinine levels are dependent on age, sex, race, and muscle mass and corrections for these factors must be used (see below). However, an *increasing* plasma creatinine over time is a red flag that there may be a renal problem.

Cystatin C levels are also dependent on age, sex, race, and muscle mass but less so than creatinine; however, cystatin C measurements alone have not been shown to be superior to formula-adjusted estimations of kidney function based on creatinine measurements, but cystatin C levels may be a useful early predictor of chronic kidney disease. Like creatinine, the elimination of cystatin C via routes other than the kidney increases with reduced GFR. Cystatin C levels can be altered in patients with cancer, thyroid dysfunction, and sometimes during glucocorticoid therapy.

It is possible to obtain a quantitative estimate of GFR based on the plasma concentration of creatinine, cystatin C, or both using formulas that have been developed over the years called eGFR equations. They include factors for age, body size, gender, and race. The age factor in the formulas accounts for the normal reduction in renal function as a person gets older. The use of any of these formulas, while subject to error, provides useful guides when obtaining a precise value for GFR is not feasible.

Finally, because urea is also handled by filtration, the same type of analysis suggests that the measurement of plasma urea concentration could also serve as an indicator of GFR. However, such a measurement is a much less accurate indicator than plasma creatinine or cystatin C because the range of normal plasma urea concentration varies widely, depending on protein intake and changes in tissue catabolism, and because urea excretion is under partial hormonal regulation.

Individual Kidney Function—Renal Scintigraphy

Clearance as described above measures the summed contribution of both kidneys. There are times when the performance of one kidney is vastly different from the other and it is necessary to assess the function of each kidney separately. This involves the injection of a radiotracer into the blood stream and then measuring the rise and fall of radioactive counts in each kidney separately using counters under each kidney, a technique called renal scintigraphy. A commonly used radioactive source is an isotope of the element technetium complexed with an organic molecule (technetium-99m mercaptoacetyltriglycine) abbreviated as MAG3. When blood containing MAG3 enters each kidney, the counts rise to a peak, and then fall in a quasi-exponential manner as the tracer is removed from the blood and moves from the renal tubules into the ureters and then bladder. A graphical plot of the activity versus time is called a *renogram*. For healthy kidneys the counts from the cortical areas reach a peak within 3 to 4 minutes, and fall with a halftime of 10 to 20 minutes. When one kidney is not performing well, this shows up as a slower rise, diminished peak level, and a flattened removal phase. To the extent that a kidney shows deficient clearance of the tracer, this indicates that it will also be deficient at clearing creatinine and other organic waste. A numerical value for MAG3 clearance by the combined kidneys can be calculated by simple regression equations from the rate at which counts arrive in the kidneys. MAG3 is cleared by the kidneys almost exclusively by secretion, and accordingly its clearance is considerably higher than creatinine clearance. Interestingly, however, MAG3 clearance and creatinine clearance are highly correlated.

KEY CONCEPTS

 Clearance expresses the rate at which a substance is removed from the plasma and excreted in the urine (renal clearance), or removed by all mechanisms combined (metabolic clearance rate), and is always quantified in units of volume per time.

 Renal clearance of any substance is calculated by a clearance formula relating urine flow to urine and plasma concentrations.

 Inulin clearance is the best measure GFR because inulin is freely filtered and neither secreted nor reabsorbed.

 Para-aminohippurate clearance can be used as an estimate of renal blood flow.

 Creatinine clearance is used as practical measure of GFR.

 Plasma creatinine concentration and/or cystatin C is used clinically as an indicator of the GFR.

 Renal scintigraphy assesses the function of each kidney separately.

STUDY QUESTIONS

3–1. We can calculate the renal clearance of any substance if we know which pair of values?

   a. Urine flow rate and urine concentration

   b. Plasma concentration and urine concentration

   c. GFR and urinary excretion rate

   d. Plasma concentration and urinary excretion rate

3–2. A drug X has a short plasma half-life and must be administered frequently to maintain therapeutic levels. The urinary concentration of X is much higher than the plasma concentration. A substantial amount of X also appears in the feces. What can we say about the renal clearance of X compared with the metabolic clearance rate of X?

   a. The metabolic clearance rate is higher than the renal clearance.

   b. The renal clearance is higher than the metabolic clearance rate.

   c. The two clearances are the same.

   d. There is insufficient information to answer the question.

3-3.   Inulin clearance is measured twice; the first time at a low inulin infusion rate, and the second time at a higher infusion rate that results in a higher plasma inulin concentration during the test. Assuming the kidneys behave the same in both cases, which measurement will yield a higher inulin clearance?

 a. The first

 b. The second

 c. Both measurements are the same.

 d. There is insufficient information to answer the question.

3-4.   Which of the following indicates correct relative renal clearances?

 a. Sodium clearance is greater than urea clearance.

 b. PAH clearance is greater than inulin clearance.

 c. Urea clearance is greater than PAH clearance.

 d. Creatinine clearance is greater than PAH clearance.

3-5.   An acute poisoning episode destroys 80% of a patient's nephrons. If the plasma urea concentration prior to the episode was 5 mmol/L, and assuming dietary protein remains the same, what is the expected value of plasma urea now?

 a. 4 mmol/L

 b. 6.25 mmol/L

 c. 25 mmol/L

 d. Continuously rising

Basic Transport Mechanisms

4

OBJECTIVES

▶ Identify the major morphological components of an epithelial tissue, including lumen, interstitium, apical and basolateral membranes, and tight junctions.

▶ State how transport mechanisms combine to achieve active transcellular reabsorption in epithelial tissues.

▶ Define iso-osmotic transport.

▶ Define paracellular transport and differentiate between transcellular and paracellular transport.

▶ Define the terms channel, transporter, uniporter, multiporter, symporter, and antiporter.

▶ Describe qualitatively the forces that determine movement of reabsorbed fluid from the interstitium into peritubular capillaries.

▶ Explain why volume reabsorption in the proximal tubule depends on activity of the Na-K-ATPase.

▶ Compare the Starling forces governing glomerular filtration with those governing peritubular capillary absorption.

▶ Compare and contrast the concepts of T_m and gradient-limited transport.

TRANSEPITHELIAL TRANSPORT

Most of the working cells of the kidneys are epithelial cells that form the walls of the renal tubules. Their task is to move a large array of substances between the lumens of the tubules and the nearby network of blood vessels. The basic process of moving these substances (secretion and reabsorption) requires that solutes and water cross the epithelium and the endothelium of the vascular walls. Substances must also traverse the thin region of interstitial fluid between them. In the cortex, where the fluxes of many filtered substances are enormous, the vascular endothelium (peritubular capillaries) is fenestrated. The fenestrae and the loose underlying basement membrane offer virtually no resistance to the passive movement of water and small solutes. This facile permeation has two consequences. First, the rate of transport between blood and tubule is governed almost exclusively by events in the tubular epithelium rather than the vascular endothelium; second, the cortical interstitium,

46

which is the medium faced by the basolateral surface of the tubular epithelia, has an osmolality and concentration of small solutes very close to those in plasma.

In contrast, both blood flow and transport events are less rapid in the medulla. Only some regions of the medullary vasculature are fenestrated, so that (1) overall transport depends on both the properties of the vascular endothelium and tubular epithelium, and (2) the medullary interstitium is most definitely *not* plasma-like in its composition. In the rest of this chapter we will describe the principles of epithelial transport that apply to all parts of the kidney, with particular emphasis on events in the cortex. We will then see how these principles apply to the medulla in subsequent chapters.

 Crossing the tubular epithelium can occur either through the cells or around the cells. The *paracellular* route is when the substance goes *around* the cells, that is, through the matrix of the tight junctions that link each epithelial cell to its neighbor. In most cases, however, a substance takes the *transcellular* route, a two-step process *through* the cells. For reabsorption, the two steps are, first, entrance across the apical membrane facing the tubular lumen, through the cell cytosol and, second, exit across the basolateral membrane facing the interstitium. For secretion the process is reversed. These structures and pathways are depicted in Figures 4–1A and B.

> ***Transcellular*** *transport: through cells—in one side and out the other;* ***paracellular*** *transport: around cells through tight junctions.*

An array of mechanisms exists by which substances cross the various barriers. These are no different from transport mechanisms used elsewhere in the body. We can view these mechanisms as a physiological tool box. Renal cells use whichever set of tools is most suitable for the task. The general classes of mechanisms for traversing the barriers are depicted in Figure 4–2.

The presence or absence of a given transport protein endows the tubular epithelium with *selectivity*, that is, the ability to choose which substance is permitted to move. Selectivity obviously applies to cell membranes containing different transport proteins (Figure 4-2A). It also applies to paracellular flux through tight junctions (Figure 4-2B). Key tight junction proteins, members of the *claudin* family, determine the degree to which various substances can travel paracellularly. In the proximal tubule, small ions like sodium and potassium, water, and urea can all move by the paracellular route. In the thick ascending limb, sodium and potassium, but not water or urea, can move paracellularly. Neither location permits the paracellular movement of glucose.

Movement by Diffusion

 Diffusion is the frenzied random movement of free molecules in solution (like the Ping-Pong balls in a lottery drawing). *Net diffusion* occurs across a barrier (i.e., more molecules moving one way than the other) if there is

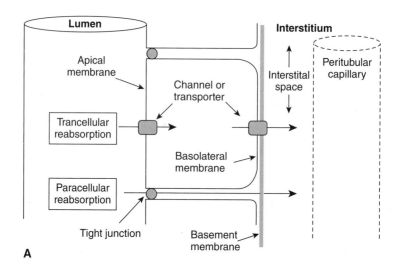

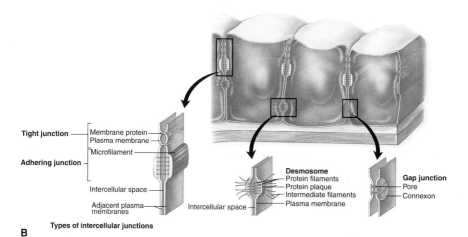

Figure 4-1. Transcellular and paracellular reabsorption (**A**) and types of intercellular junctions (**B**). Transcellular reabsorption is a two-step process with separate influx and efflux steps utilizing transporters or channels. Paracellular reabsorption is always a passive process through the tight junctions. (Reproduced with permission from McKinley M, O'Loughlin VD. *Human Anatomy*, 2nd ed. New York: McGraw-Hill, 2008.)

driving force (a concentration gradient or, for charged molecules, a potential gradient) and if the barrier is permeable. Movement by net diffusion applies to almost all substances crossing the endothelial barrier lining the peritubular capillaries. It also applies to substances taking the paracellular route around the tubular epithelium and to some substances taking the transcellular route through membranes. Small neutral molecules that are lipid soluble, such as the blood gases, alcohol, and steroids, can diffuse directly through the lipid bilayer.

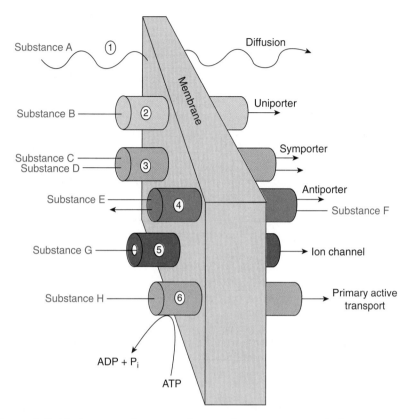

Figure 4–2. Mechanisms of transmembrane solute transport. With the exception of simple diffusion through the lipid bilayer, all transport involves channels and transporters that are regulated by signaling pathways.

Movement Through Channels

Most substances of biological importance cannot penetrate lipid membranes fast enough to meet cellular needs. To speed up the process their transmembrane flux is mediated by integral membrane proteins, which are divided into categories of *channels* and *transporters* (see Figure 4–2). Channels are small pores (proteins with a "hole" through the interior of the protein) that permit, depending on their structure, water or specific solutes to diffuse through them. Thus, we use the terms *sodium channel* and *potassium channel* to designate proteins that permit diffusion of these molecular species. *Aquaporins* are channels that permit the diffusion of water. Some species of aquaporin also permit diffusion of small neutral molecules including carbon dioxide (CO_2) and nitric oxide (NO). Channels typically flicker open and closed like camera shutters so that the permeability of a membrane containing many channels is proportional to the number of channels and the probability of their being open. Movement through channels is passive, that is, no external energy is required. The energy to drive the diffusion is inherent in the

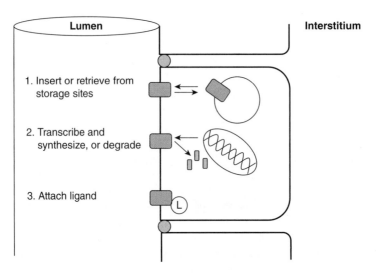

Figure 4–3. Common mechanisms for regulating channel and transporter activity. 1. Transport proteins are shuttled back and forth between the surface membrane, where they function normally, and sites of sequestration at the base of microvilli or in intracellular vesicles. 2. Transport protein is synthesized and inserted in the membrane, or removed and degraded. 3. Transport proteins are activated or inhibited by attaching ligands, either covalently (e.g., phosphorylation) or reversibly (e.g., ATP).

concentration gradient or, strictly speaking, the electrochemical gradient, because charged ions are driven through channels and around cells via the paracellular route not only by gradients of concentration but also by gradients of voltage. Channels represent a mechanism for rapid movement of specific substances across membranes, which would otherwise diffuse slowly or not at all.

A characteristic of channels critical for renal function is the regulation of their permeability by a number of environmental factors and signaling cascades (Figure 4–3). First, many channel types can be *gated*, meaning that the probability that the channel is open can be increased or decreased. The topic of channel gating is a whole story by itself, but several ways of gating channels include reversible binding of small molecules that are components of signaling cascades (ligand-gated channels), changes in membrane potential (voltage-gated channels), and mechanical distortion (stretch-gated channels). Second, many channel types have phosphorylation sites such that phosphorylation either locks the channel shut or allows it to be gated by one of the mechanisms above. Third, some channel species can be moved back and forth between the surface membrane and intracellular vesicles, thereby regulating how many of the existing channels are actually functioning as permeability pathways. Finally, and on a slower time scale, the genomic expression of channels is regulated so that the total number of channels, whether in the membrane or sequestered in vesicles, is altered up or down. Channel and transporter proteins are not permanent fixtures in the membrane. Their lifetimes in the membrane are generally in the range of a few hours. All of these regulatory processes are controlled by intricate signaling cascades that are the subject of much current research.

Movement by Transporters

Our genome codes for a large array of proteins that function as transporters, all with names and acronyms that suffuse the physiological literature. Transporters, like channels, permit the transmembrane flux of a solute that is otherwise impermeable in the lipid bilayer. Channels can move large amounts of materials across membranes in a short period of time, but most transporters have a lower rate of transport because the transported solutes bind much more strongly to the transport protein. Furthermore, the protein must undergo a more elaborate cycle of conformational change to move the solute from one side of the membrane to the other. However, overall flux rate depends not only on the kinetics of individual transporters, but also on the density of transporters in the membrane. Total flux via transporters can be very high if the transporter density is high. As is the case for channels, the amount of substance moved via transporters is highly regulated. The regulation includes changes in phosphorylation of the transporter (thereby turning its activity on or off), sequestration into vesicles, and of course changes in genomic expression. As described next, we group transporters into categories according to basic functional properties.

UNIPORTERS

Uniporters permit movement of a single solute species through the membrane. The basic difference between a channel and a uniporter is that a channel is a tiny hole, whereas a uniporter requires that the solute bind to a site that is alternately available to one side and then the other side of the membrane (like entering a vestibule with a turnstile through an outside door, passing through the turnstile, and then leaving the vestibule to enter a hallway through an inside door). Movement through a uniporter is often called *facilitated diffusion* because, like diffusion, it is driven by concentration gradients, but the transported solute moves through the uniporter protein rather than the membrane lipid. A set of uniporters crucial for all cells includes those that facilitate the movement of glucose across cell membranes. These are members of the GLUT family of proteins that permit, in the kidney's proximal tubule epithelial cells, glucose to move from the cytosol across the basolateral membrane into the interstitium. Another uniporter family important for renal function is the UT family that transports urea. We will see in Chapter 6 how this family plays a role in regulating renal water excretion.

MULTIPORTERS: SYMPORTERS AND ANTIPORTERS

Multiporters move two or more solute species across a membrane simultaneously. Symporters move them together in the same direction. Antiporters move them in opposite directions. In the literature, symporters are sometimes called *cotransporters*, and antiporters are called *exchangers*. Important symporters for the handling of glucose move sodium and glucose together into cells (members of the SGLT protein family). Each transport cycle moves one glucose molecule and either one or

> *Channels are holes; transporters bind solutes and then move them by changing conformation.*

two sodium ions depending on the particular species of SGLT. Another key symporter in the kidney is one that moves sodium, potassium, and chloride all together into a cell (Na-K-2Cl). Important antiporters in the kidneys (and many other organs) move sodium into a cell and protons out of a cell (often called sodium-hydrogen exchangers, members of the NHE protein family). Yet another family of antiporters in many cells, including the kidney, moves chloride in one direction and bicarbonate in the opposite direction. In later chapters we will see how these and other transporters play defined roles in specific nephron segments.

All molecular transport requires energy. In the case of diffusion through a channel or movement via a uniporter, the energy is inherent in the electrochemical gradient of the solute. With symporters and antiporters, at least one of the solutes moves down its electrochemical gradient and provides the energy to move one or more of the other solutes up its electrochemical gradient (like a pulley system where a small weight is raised by the downward movement of a heavier weight on the other side of the pulley). Movement of any solute up its electrochemical gradient is called *active transport*. In the case of symporters and antiporters that do not hydrolyze ATP, the active transport is called *secondary* active transport because the energy is provided indirectly from the transport of another solute rather than directly from a chemical reaction. In a large number of cases, sodium is one of the solutes moved by a symporter or antiporter. The electrochemical gradient of sodium in all cells favors entrance. *Passive* movement of sodium is therefore always inward. When sodium movement is coupled to that of another solute, as in sodium-proton antiport (exchange), sodium will normally enter. The stoichiometry is important here. The energy available from a gradient is multiplied by the number of molecules that move per transport cycle. For example, sodium/calcium antiporters move three sodium ions per calcium ion. Calcium has a larger electrochemical gradient than does sodium, but this difference is overcome by moving three sodium ions per cycle of the antiporter.

Another example where the stoichiometry plays an essential role is the coupled transport of bicarbonate and sodium. An important symporter in the proximal tubule is the NBCe transporter, which moves three bicarbonate ions and one sodium ion out of the cell per transport cycle. The electrochemical gradient for bicarbonate is directly outward, and the energy gained from moving three bicarbonate ions outward is greater than the energy it takes to move one sodium ion outward against its electrochemical gradient. Therefore, this transporter moves both solutes outward, *up* the electrochemical gradient for sodium. This is a rare case of sodium removal by something other than an ATPase.

PRIMARY ACTIVE TRANSPORTERS

Primary active transporters are membrane proteins that move one or more solutes up their electrochemical gradients, using the energy obtained from the hydrolysis of adenosine triphosphate (ATP). All transporters that move solutes in this manner are ATPases, that is, their structure is both that of an enzyme that splits ATP and a transporter that has binding sites that alternately are open to one side and then the other side of the membrane. Among the key primary active transporters in the kidney is the ubiquitous Na-K-ATPase, often called the "sodium pump," some isoform of which is present in virtually all cells of the body. This transporter simultaneously moves sodium against its electrochemical gradient out of a cell and potassium against its gradient into a cell. The stoichiometry is three sodium ions out and two potassium ions for each ATP molecule hydrolyzed. Other crucial primary active transport systems are H-ATPases, which move protons out of cells, and Ca-ATPases, which move calcium out of cells. All of these ATPases belong to a large family of homologous transporter proteins. Yet another important class of primary active transporters are the multidrug resistance proteins (MDR, also called ATP-binding cassette proteins), named for their ability to remove therapeutic drugs from cells. Unlike the inorganic ion ATPases, which are quite selective for the ion species they move, the MDR transporters unselectively transport a wide variety of organic anions.

RECEPTOR-MEDIATED ENDOCYTOSIS AND TRANSCYTOSIS

Almost all the secretion and reabsorption of solutes discussed throughout this textbook use some combination of the just-mentioned set of membrane permeability mechanisms. One other solute transport process of some importance is *receptor-mediated endocytosis*. In this case, a solute, usually a protein, binds to a site on the apical surface of an epithelial cell, and then a patch of membrane with the solute bound to it is internalized as a vesicle in the cytoplasm. Subsequent processes then degrade the protein into its constituent amino acids, which are transported across the basolateral membrane and into the blood.

For a few proteins, particularly immunoglobulins, endocytosis can occur at either the apical or basolateral membranes, after which the endocytic vesicles remain intact and are transported to the opposite cellular membrane, where they undergo exocytosis to release the protein intact. Such *transcytosis* is very important in the host defense mechanisms of the kidney and in the prevention of urinary tract infections.

Osmosis and Osmotic Pressure

OSMOTIC VOCABULARY

The vocabulary of osmotic matters is often used loosely, leading to some confusion, but the central concept is straightforward. Solutes dissolved in water displace some of the water and lower its concentration. Therefore solutions differing in solute concentration also differ in water concentration. Given the opportunity to do so, water diffuses from where its concentration is higher (dilute solutions) into solutions where its concentration is lower (concentrated solutions), a process called *osmosis*.

Dissolved solutes that displace water are called *osmoles*. One mole of any dissolved solute (an Avogadro's number of it; about 6.02×10^{23}) is one osmole. The sum of the moles in a mixture gives us the total number of osmoles. For example, one-half mole of urea and one-half mole of sucrose together make one total osmole. Since salts dissociate in solution, one mole of salt molecules that splits into two ions (e.g., NaCl) becomes two osmoles, and a mole of salt that splits into three ions (e.g., $CaCl_2$) becomes three osmoles.

The concentration of osmoles is expressed by the terms osmolarity and osmolality. *Osmolarity* is the number of osmoles per liter of solution, most commonly it is expressed in "milli" units (mOsm/L). A solution containing 50 mM urea and 100 mM NaCl has an osmolarity of 250 mOsm/L (50 urea, 100 Na^+ and 100 Cl^-). Osmolarity is a convenient unit because we can easily calculate it from the known ingredients in solution. *Osmolality* is the concentration of osmoles per kilogram of water, for example, 300 mOsM/kg H_2O. Since a liter of solution contains almost 1 kg of water, the values of osmolarity and osmolality are nearly the same.

All of the above assumes that solutions are *ideal* (i.e., any dissolved solute particle is the same as any other and is fully active osmotically), but real solutions are not ideal. Solutes interact with each other in mysterious ways such that a mole of most solutes, when dissolved, results in less than one osmole. It is the *real* osmolality that determines the movement of water between fluid compartments. These concepts are illustrated in the case of physiological saline (0.9% NaCl, or 154 mmol/L NaCl). This solution is commonly used as a hospital infusion solution because it matches the normal osmolality of human plasma (280–290 mOsm/kg H_2O). The osmolarity of this solution, assuming ideality, is $154 + 154 = 308$ mOsm/L, but the measured osmolality is 287 mOsm/kg H_2O. Any solution with the same real osmolality as normal human plasma is said to be an *isosmotic* solution. For convenience, physiologists often calculate osmolarity assuming the solution to be ideal and then *call it* osmolality, and accept the error in this calculation as the price paid for convenience.

Osmotic pressure is another confusing concept. Despite its name, osmotic pressure is not a pressure in the sense of hydrostatic pressure—it just means osmolality. A beaker of water and a beaker of glucose solution with a high osmolality both have the same hydrostatic pressure at any level of depth, but different osmotic pressures. By definition osmotic pressure is the pressure that theoretically would have to be applied to a solution to prevent the movement of water by osmosis across a semipermeable barrier from pure water into the solution. (A semipermeable barrier is permeable to water, but not solute). Numerically it is the just real osmolality expressed in pressure units. This equivalence is expressed by the van't Hoff equation, where π is the osmotic pressure, R and T are the gas constant and absolute temperature, and C is the osmolality (osmolarity is usually used as an approximation for osmolality).

$$\pi = RTC$$

To calculate a numerical value for osmotic pressure in units of mm Hg, multiply the osmolality by 19.3. Thus an osmolality difference of only 1 mOsm/kg H_2O is actually a significant driving force for the movement of water.

WATER MOVEMENT ACROSS SEMIPERMEABLE BARRIERS

 If the solutions on either side of a semipermeable barrier differ in osmolality, water moves by osmosis toward the solution with the higher osmolality. Although water is driven by its own concentration gradient, it is convenient to think of solute as "pulling" water. The kidneys make use of this concept by reabsorbing solutes across the renal tubules (from lumen to the interstitium) and allowing water to follow, that is, "water follows the osmoles." Differences in osmolality are only effective in driving osmosis when the barrier is less permeable to solutes than to water, that is, it is semipermeable. (Imagine a barrier made of chicken wire. Regardless of osmolalities, there would be no osmosis because there would be no restriction on the diffusion of solute.)

> *Water is transported by "following the osmoles."*

 In the fenestrated endothelial barriers of glomerular capillaries and peritubular capillaries, most of the solutes are as permeable through the fenestrae as water and thus do not influence water movement. However, the large plasma proteins are not permeable, and they do indeed influence water movement. The osmotic pressure resulting from the proteins only (ignoring everything else) is called the *colloid osmotic pressure* or *oncotic pressure*. Colloid osmotic pressure is a component of the Starling forces governing filtration and absorption across endothelial layers. In other barriers, specifically the epithelial lining of the renal tubules, the permeabilities of all solutes are generally lower than water permeability. Therefore, all solutes contribute to driving a water flux. Here, *all* of the osmolality, not just the component resulting from proteins, is important.

PROXIMAL TUBULE REABSORPTION

Virtually all of the 180 L of water and several pounds of salt and other solutes filtered each day into Bowman's space are reabsorbed, along with large amounts of many other substances. Most of this reabsorption occurs in the proximal tubule. Almost all solutes (except large plasma proteins) are filtered from plasma into Bowman's space in the same proportion as water; thus, their concentrations in the glomerular filtrate are the same as in the plasma. By the end of the proximal tubule about two-thirds of the water and solutes have been reabsorbed. The rates of reabsorption, and thus concentrations in the lumen at the end of the proximal tubule, vary from solute to solute, but the summed total of solutes (osmoles) reabsorbed is proportional to water reabsorbed. This is called iso-osmotic reabsorption. In the later portions of the nephron, beyond the proximal tubule, reabsorption is generally not iso-osmotic, meaning that water and total solute reabsorption are usually not proportional. This is crucial for our ability to independently regulate solute and water balance.

Sodium and Water

Sodium accounts for nearly half of the total solute load appearing in the glomerular filtrate, and most of the rest consists of the anions (primarily chloride and bicarbonate) that must accompany sodium to maintain electroneutrality. Similarly, sodium and its accompanying anions account for the vast majority of solutes reabsorbed in the proximal tubule. The large amount of sodium and anions transferred from lumen to interstitium sets up an osmotic gradient that favors the parallel movement of

> In the proximal tubule the transport of water and every solute is tied directly or indirectly to the active transport of sodium by the Na-K-ATPase.

water. The proximal tubule epithelium is very permeable to water, which follows the osmoles across in equal proportions. Thus both the fluid removed from the lumen and that remaining behind are essentially iso-osmotic with the original filtrate. We say "essentially" because there must be *some* difference in osmolality to induce water movement, but for an epithelial barrier like the proximal tubule that is very permeable to water, a difference of less than 1 mOsm/kg is sufficient to drive reabsorption of water. (Recall that an osmolality difference of 1 mOsM/kg is equal in driving force to 19.3 mm Hg of hydrostatic pressure.) Once in the interstitium, the solutes and water move from interstitium into the peritubular capillaries and are returned to the systemic circulation (Table 4–1).

Epithelial transport requires that the cells be *polarized*, that is, the proteins present in the apical and the basolateral membranes are not the same. In the case of sodium, polarization of the proximal tubule epithelium promotes net flux from lumen to interstitium. Movement of sodium is the linchpin around which

Table 4–1. Estimated forces involved in the movement of fluid from interstitium into peritubular capillaries*

Forces	mm Hg
1. Favoring uptake	
a. Interstitial hydraulic pressure, P_{Int}	3
b. Oncotic pressure in peritubular capillaries, π_{PC}	33
2. Opposing uptake	
a. Hydraulic pressure in peritubular capillaries, P_{PC}	20
b. Interstitial oncotic pressure, π_{Int}	6
3. Net pressure for uptake (1–2)	10

*The values for peritubular-capillary hydraulic and oncotic pressures are for the early portions of the capillary. The oncotic pressure, of course, decreases as protein-free fluid enters it (i.e., as absorption occurs) but would not go below 25 mm Hg (the value of arterial plasma) even if all fluid originally filtered at the glomerulus were absorbed.

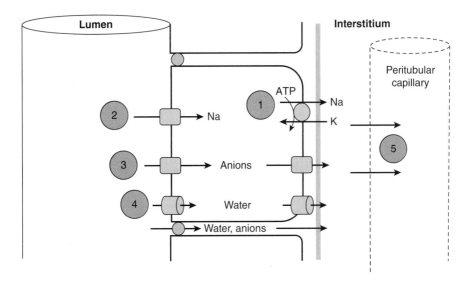

Figure 4–4. Epithelial salt and water reabsorption. See text for explanation of each individual step.

the transport of virtually every other substance depends. Figure 4–4 shows the morphology of a generalized proximal tubule epithelium in which salt and water transport can be viewed as a multistep process.

Step 1 is the active extrusion of sodium from epithelial cell to interstitium across the basolateral membrane. Step 2 is the passive entrance of sodium from the tubular lumen across the apical membrane into the cell to replace the sodium removed in step 1. Step 3 is the parallel movement of anions from lumen to interstitium that must accompany the sodium to preserve electroneutrality. Step 4 is the osmotic flow of water from tubular lumen to interstitium. Finally, step 5 is the bulk flow of water and salt from interstitium into the peritubular capillary. Let us examine these steps more closely.

The active extrusion of sodium in step 1 is via the Na-K-ATPase, which is the major energy consumer in the cell. The action of the Na-K-ATPase has several consequences, the key one being that it keeps the concentration of sodium within the cell low enough to favor the passive entrance of sodium from lumen to cell in all the processes of step 2.

The entrance of sodium into the cell in step 2 is via multiple pathways. Quantitatively most of sodium enters via the sodium-proton antiporter (NHE3 isoform). As we will see later, regulation of this transporter is a key player in regulating sodium excretion.

Step 3, the movement of anions, is the most complex, as it involves two ions (chloride and bicarbonate) and a variety of transcellular and paracellular processes. We will examine the details later, but for now we emphasize that the movement of sodium, which is a cation, must be matched quantitatively by the equal movement of anions.

Step 4 is the osmotic movement of water. The tubular cells possess a complement of aquaporins in both the apical and basolateral membranes, and the tight junctions are also permeable to water. Therefore, as steps 1 to 3 lower the local luminal osmotic concentration by even a few milliosmoles per liter, water flows osmotically from lumen to interstitium.

The movement of water into the interstitium in step 4 promotes step 5. This is the bulk flow of fluid from interstitium to peritubular capillary driven by Starling forces (hydrostatic and oncotic pressure gradients). The capillary hydraulic pressure by itself opposes the uptake of interstitial fluids, but its value of 15 to 20 mm Hg is much lower than the 60 mm Hg in the glomerular capillaries, where there is net filtration. Meanwhile, the plasma oncotic pressure has risen to more than 30 mm Hg because loss of water by filtration in the glomerular capillaries concentrates the large plasma proteins. There is also a small but significant, interstitial pressure. The sum of these Starling forces is a net absorptive pressure, and it drives fluid movement into the peritubular capillaries. The reader can appreciate the fact that if cortical Starling forces are abnormal (e.g., low plasma oncotic pressure as when liver disease prevents normal production of serum albumin), absorption of fluid from the cortical interstitium can be slowed, causing a backup of fluid that inhibits fluid movement from tubular lumen to interstitium. Ultimately, this can lead to increased excretion of water and electrolytes from the body.

> *Water reabsorption in the proximal tubule concentrates all the remaining unreabsorbed solutes.*

Consequences for Other Solutes

The events just described have consequences for all the other solutes filtered along with sodium and its anions. As water follows sodium and its anions across the epithelium, the luminal volume decreases, thereby concentrating all remaining solutes. If two-thirds of the water is removed, any solute not previously removed will increase in concentration by a factor of 3. As its luminal concentration rises, this generates a concentration gradient across the tight junctions between the lumen and the interstitium. (The interstitial concentration of transported substances is essentially clamped to the plasma value because of the high peritubular blood flow and high permeability of the fenestrated capillaries.) If the tight junctions are permeable to the substance in question ("leaky"), the substance diffuses from the lumen to the interstitium, and then into the peritubular capillaries along with sodium and water. This is precisely what happens to many solutes (e.g., urea, potassium, calcium, and magnesium) in the proximal tubule. The exact fractions of the filtered load that are reabsorbed depend on the permeability of the tight junctions, but are generally in the range of one-half to two-thirds. As indicated earlier, one substance that does *not* move by the paracellular route is glucose, which is impermeable in the tight junctions. We will describe the fate of filtered glucose in Chapter 5.

Limits on Rate of Transport: T_m and Gradient-Limited Systems

Even though the transport capacity of the renal tubules is huge, it is not infinite. There are upper limits to the rate at which any given solute can be reabsorbed or secreted. In situations in which unusually large amounts of a substance are filtered, these limits are reached, with the consequence that larger than normal amounts of solute are *not* reabsorbed (i.e., left in the lumen and passed on to the next nephron segment). In general, transport mechanisms can be classified by the properties of these limits as either (1) tubular maximum-limited (T_m) systems or (2) gradient-limited systems.

The classification is based on the leakiness of the tight junctions. Consider first gradient-limited systems. When the tight junctions are very leaky to a given substance, for example sodium, it is impossible for the removal of the substance from the lumen to reduce its luminal concentration very much below that in the cortical interstitium. As the substance is removed and the luminal concentration starts to fall, the gradient between these two media increases, causing the substance to leak back as fast as it is removed (like bailing a very leaky boat). Thus, for sodium and all other substances whose reabsorption is characterized by a gradient-limited system, the luminal concentration remains close to the interstitial concentration. Be aware that the existence of a limiting rate does not stop reabsorption in normal circumstances because water is being reabsorbed simultaneously. Even though the luminal *concentration* does not decrease very much, large amounts are still being removed. In contrast, if unusual osmotic conditions retard water reabsorption, then removal of the substance is not accompanied by a corresponding amount of water. Consequently, reabsorption reduces the luminal concentration and the limiting gradient is indeed reached. Now the substance leaks back, leaving unusually high amounts of the substance in the large volume of unreabsorbed water.

> *The rate of reabsorption for any substance is limited by the capacity of the transporters (T_m systems) or by paracellular back leak (gradient-limited).*

Now consider T_m-limited systems. In this case the tight junctions are *impermeable* to the solutes in question. There is no back leak and no limit on the size of the difference in concentration between lumen and interstitium. The limit on transport rate instead is due to the capacity of the transporters to remove the substance (the inherent kinetic properties of the transport proteins and their density in the membrane). As the filtered load rises, the amount reabsorbed increases in parallel, up to the point of saturating the transporters. For loads below the T_m, virtually all is reabsorbed. But any increase in filtered load above the T_m does not increase transport out of the lumen. Consequently the excess is left behind. In most cases, the amount that escapes reabsorption in the proximal tubule is excreted.

The functional reasons for differentiating between T_m and gradient-limited systems is that solutes handled by T_m systems will, if the filtered load is below the T_m, be reabsorbed essentially completely, whereas solutes handled by gradient-limited systems are *never* reabsorbed completely, that is, a substantial amount always remains in the tubule to be passed on to the next nephron segment.

Osmotic Diuresis

If the normal tight coupling between sodium and water reabsorption in the proximal tubule is disrupted, we have a phenomenon known as *osmotic diuresis.* The term diuresis simply means increased urine flow, and *osmotic* diuresis denotes the situation in which the increased urine flow is due to an abnormally high amount of any solute that is not reabsorbed at all (e.g., mannitol) or is filtered at such a high rate that much is left in the tubule (e.g., very high plasma glucose), leaving large amounts of solute (osmoles) in the lumen. As water is reabsorbed from the tubule, the concentration of any unreabsorbed solute rises. Its osmotic presence retards the further reabsorption of water, that is, it is "holding" water in the lumen. If this occurs in the proximal tubule it also retards net sodium reabsorption. Why is that? Sodium transport per se continues unabated. But since water is being held in the lumen, the sodium transport causes an initial fall in luminal sodium concentration. This then drives a passive back leak of sodium via tight junctions because the limiting gradient for sodium transport is reached. At this point there is little *net* sodium transport because the amount reabsorbed is matched by the amount leaking back. The result is that high amounts of sodium, water, and the unusual solute pass on to the loop of Henle. Osmotic diuresis can occur in persons with uncontrolled diabetes mellitus in which the filtered load of glucose exceeds the tubular maximum (T_m), and the unreabsorbed glucose then acts as an osmotic diuretic. In other cases it can be due to an infused solute such as mannitol that is filtered, but not transported at all.

KEY CONCEPTS

Flux from lumen to interstitium can be transcellular, using separate transport steps in the apical and basolateral membranes, or paracellular, around the cells through tight junctions.

The kidneys move solutes across membranes by multiple transport mechanisms, including channels, uniporters, multiporters, and primary active transporters.

The kidneys regulate excretion by regulating channels and transporters in epithelial cell membranes.

Water crosses epithelial barriers by movement down osmotic gradients (from regions of lower to higher osmolality).

 Volume reabsorption is a multistep process involving transport across epithelial membranes from lumen to interstitium, and bulk flow from interstitium to peritubular capillaries driven by Starling forces.

 The reabsorption of water concentrates all remaining tubular solutes, increasing the driving force for their passive reabsorption by diffusion.

 All reabsorptive processes have a limit on how fast they can occur, either because the substance leaks back into the lumen (gradient-limited systems) or because the transporters saturate (T_m systems).

STUDY QUESTIONS

4–1. A healthy patient has a normal plasma osmolality (close to 300 mOsm/kg). If 100 mmol of solutes are reabsorbed iso-osmotically from the proximal tubule, approximately how much water is reabsorbed with the solute?

    a. 100 mL

    b. 300 mL

    c. 333 mL

    d. 1000 mL

4–2. Quantitatively, most sodium enters proximal tubule cells by:

    a. paracellular diffusion.

    b. transcellular diffusion.

    c. the Na-K-ATPase.

    d. antiport with hydrogen ions.

4–3. The tight junctions linking proximal tubule cells permit passive diffusion of:

    a. glucose.

    b. sodium.

    c. all filtered solutes.

    d. no filtered solutes.

4–4. In the proximal tubule, water can move through

    a. apical membranes of proximal tubule cells.

    b. basolateral membranes of proximal tubule cells.

    c. tight junctions.

    d. all of these.

4–5. A drug X is secreted into the proximal tubule by a T_m-limited system. This implies that:

    a. X cannot easily diffuse by the paracellular route.

    b. all the X that enters the renal vasculature will be secreted.

    c. the rate of X secretion is independent of the plasma concentration.

    d. X is not filtered at the glomerulus.

4–6. All multiporters do what?

    a. Simultaneously move several molecules of a given solute (e.g., three sodium ions or two glucose molecules).

    b. Simultaneously move two or more different solute species.

    c. Use ATP to energize the transport.

    d. Move transported solutes in the same direction.

Renal Handling of Organic Solutes

5

OBJECTIVES

▶ State the physiological utility of either excreting or reabsorbing organic solutes.
▶ State the general characteristics of the proximal tubular systems for active reabsorption or secretion of organic nutrients.
▶ Describe the renal handling of glucose and state the conditions under which glycosuria is likely to occur.
▶ Describe the renal handling of proteins and small peptides.
▶ Describe the secretion of para-aminohippurate.
▶ Outline the handling of urate.
▶ Describe the secretion of organic cations.
▶ Describe how tubular pH affects the excretion and reabsorption of weak acids and bases.
▶ Describe the renal handling of urea, including the medullary recycling of urea from the collecting duct to the loop of Henle.

OVERVIEW

As pointed out in Chapter 1, a major function of the kidneys is the excretion of organic waste, foreign chemicals, and their metabolites. As the kidneys excrete these substances they also filter large amounts of organic substances that they do *not* excrete, such as glucose and amino acids. Therefore the kidneys must discriminate between what to keep and what to discard. While the collective concentration of the useful organic solutes that should be kept is small in comparison with inorganic ions like sodium and chloride, the large amounts filtered means that processes must exist to reabsorb them.

Some organic solutes handled by the kidneys are neutral molecules; most are anions or cations. As the useful metabolites are recovered from the filtrate; the waste and foreign substances are not only let go, but actively secreted. Since most of these solutes are predominantly protein-bound, secretion represents the major route by which they enter the tubule. In dealing with organic solutes the kidneys perform a kind of triage. They (1) reabsorb metabolites that should be retained, glucose being the obvious example, (2) eliminate waste products, uremic toxins, and foreign substances, and (3) partially reabsorb a few special solutes. An analysis of the renal handling of every one of these organic substances would be prohibitive, so we will discuss a few key solutes and establish generalities about the others.

One organic substance, urea, is unique in this regard. It is a waste product that must be excreted to prevent accumulation. However, it also plays a key role in renal regulation of water balance. The renal handling of urea is briefly discussed later in this chapter and again in the following chapter in the discussion of renal handling of water.

General Properties of Organic Solute Transport

 Several generalizations apply to the handling of small organic solutes by the kidney.

1. While there is a strikingly large number of organic solute species, there is a far smaller number of transport protein species, meaning that many transporters are promiscuous, accepting multiple solutes, sometimes over 100 different ones. This allows the kidneys to operate without expressing a separate transporter for each and every solute.
2. Most organic solutes are transported *only* in the proximal tubule. Those that are secreted or escape reabsorption in the proximal tubule end up being excreted (an exception, as covered later in this chapter, is when charged species become neutral as a result of changes in tubular pH and are reabsorbed passively in regions beyond the proximal tubule).
3. Transport involves a cascade of interrelated transport events always beginning with active extrusion of sodium across the basolateral membrane of proximal tubule cells by the Na-K-ATPase. Neutral or negatively charged organic solutes then enter via symporters with sodium, while cations enter via uniporters driven by the negative membrane potential. The resulting intracellular accumulation of the solute in question establishes a favorable gradient for its efflux. The accumulated solutes then leave through a variety of pathways across the opposite membrane from which they entered, or couple via an antiporter to the influx of another organic solute.

> *Organic solutes are transported only in the proximal tubule (urea is an exception).*

PROXIMAL REABSORPTION OF ORGANIC NUTRIENTS

Most of the useful organic nutrients in the plasma that should not be lost in the urine are freely filtered. These include glucose, amino acids, acetate, Krebs cycle intermediates, some water-soluble vitamins, lactate, acetoacetate, β-hydroxybutyrate, and many others. The proximal tubule is the major site for reabsorption of the large quantities of these organic nutrients filtered each day by the renal corpuscles.

Glucose

 Under most circumstances, it would be deleterious to lose glucose in the urine, particularly in conditions of prolonged fasting. Thus the kidneys normally reabsorb all the glucose that is filtered. A typical plasma glucose level is about 90 mg/dL (5 mmol/L). It rises transiently to well over 100 mg/dL during meals and falls somewhat during fasting. Usually all the filtered glucose is reabsorbed in the proximal tubule. This involves taking up glucose from the tubular lumen across the apical membrane via sodium-glucose symporters, followed by its exit across the basolateral membrane into the interstitium via a GLUT uniporter. Most of the glucose is reabsorbed by a high capacity, low affinity sodium-glucose symporter (SGLT-2) that has a stoichiometry of one sodium per glucose. Then the last remaining glucose is taken up in the late proximal tubule (S3 segment) by a low capacity, high affinity transporter (SGLT-1) that transports two sodium ions per glucose (Figure 5–1 top). This two-for-one stoichiometry provides additional energy to move glucose up its concentration gradient in the region where the luminal concentration has already been greatly reduced. Unlike the case for sodium and many other solutes, the tight junctions are not significantly permeable to glucose. Therefore, as glucose is removed from the lumen and the luminal concentration falls, there is no back-leak, resulting in virtually complete reabsorption.

Because the sodium-glucose symporters are saturable (T_m system systems), abnormally high filtered loads overwhelm the reabsorptive capacity (exceed the T_m; Figure 5–1 bottom). This occurs when plasma glucose approaches 200 mg/dL, a situation often found in untreated diabetes mellitus. In very severe cases plasma glucose can exceed 1000 mg/dL, or over 55 mmol/L, leading to significant loss of glucose.

If we assume that the T_m for glucose transport is 375 mg/min (a typical value), glomerular filtration rate (GFR) is 125 mL/min (1.25 dL/min) and plasma glucose is a normal 90 mg/dL, the filtered load is 1.25 dL/min × 90 mg/dL = 112.5 mg/min. This is well below the T_m of 375 mg/min. Thus the kidneys easily reabsorb the entire filtered load. When plasma glucose reaches 200 mg/dL, the filtered load is now 1.25 dL/min × 200 mg/dL = 250 mg/min. At this point, some individual nephrons have reached the upper limit of what they can reabsorb, and a little glucose begins to spill into the urine. Further increases in plasma glucose saturate the remaining transporters and any amount filtered above 375 mg/min is excreted. This leads to loss of glucose and an unwanted osmotic diuresis that we discussed in Chapter 4. One can appreciate that any glucose not reabsorbed is an osmole in the tubule that has consequences for water reabsorption.

Recently, the FDA has approved a class of SGLT-2 inhibitors (the glyflozins) that lead to excretion of a large fraction of the filtered load of glucose. They are very useful for treating type 2 diabetes, particularly in its early stages, and can substantially reduce blood glucose. As we would expect from our consideration of osmotic diuresis, the drugs do increase urine volume.

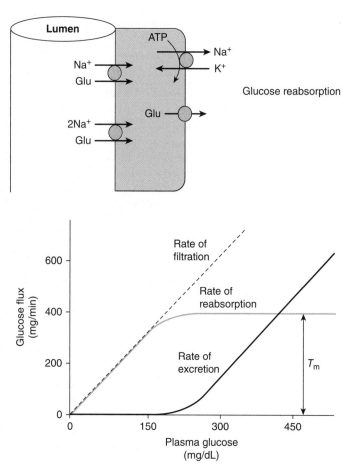

Figure 5–1. Glucose handling by the kidney. (Top) Glucose is taken up across the apical membrane by sodium-glucose symporters and leaves across the basolateral membrane via glucose uniporters (GLUT family). In most of the proximal tubule the sodium-glucose stoichiometry is one-for-one (SGLT-2 isoform). In the late proximal tubule the stoichiometry is two-for-one (SGLT-1 isoform). (Bottom) The rates of filtration, reabsorption, and excretion are plotted as a function of plasma glucose concentration. At a given GFR, the rate of glucose filtration is exactly proportional to the plasma concentration. At normal levels of plasma glucose this rate is well below the T_m, and therefore all the filtered glucose is reabsorbed and none is excreted. However, as plasma glucose rises into the hyperglycemic range, the T_m is reached and any glucose filtered in excess of the T_m is excreted.

PROTEINS AND PEPTIDES

 Although we sometimes say the glomerular filtrate is protein free, it is not truly free of all protein; it just has a total protein concentration much lower than plasma. First, peptides and smaller proteins (e.g., angiotensin, insulin), although present at low concentrations in the blood, are filtered in considerable quantities. Second, while the movement of large plasma proteins across the glomerular filtration barrier is extremely limited, a small amount does make it through into Bowman's space. For albumin, the plasma protein of highest concentration in the blood, the concentration in the filtrate is normally about 1 mg/dL, or roughly 0.02% of the plasma albumin concentration (5 g/dL). But due to the huge volume of fluid filtered per day, the total filtered amount of protein is not negligible. Normally all of these proteins and peptides are reabsorbed completely, although not in the conventional way. They are enzymatically degraded into their constituent amino acids, which are then returned to the blood.

For the larger proteins, the initial step in recovery is endocytosis at the apical membrane. This energy-requiring process is triggered by the binding of filtered protein molecules to specific receptors on the apical membrane. The rate of endocytosis is increased in proportion to the concentration of protein in the glomerular filtrate until a maximal rate of vesicle formation, and thus the T_m for protein uptake, is reached. The pinched-off intracellular vesicles resulting from endocytosis merge with lysosomes, whose enzymes degrade the protein to low-molecular-weight fragments, mainly individual amino acids. These end products then exit the cells across the basolateral membrane into the interstitial fluid, from which they gain entry to the peritubular capillaries.

To understand the potential problem associated with a failure to take up filtered protein, remember that for a healthy young adult

$$\text{Total filtered protein} = \text{GFR} \times \text{concentration of protein in filtrate}$$
$$= 180\text{L/day} \times 10 \text{ mg/L} = 1.8 \text{ g/day} \qquad \text{Equation 5-1}$$

If this protein was not removed from the lumen, the entire 1.8 g would be lost in the urine. In fact, most of the filtered protein is endocytosed and degraded so that the excretion of protein in the urine is normally only 100 mg/day. The endocytic mechanism by which protein is taken up is easily saturated, so a large increase in filtered protein resulting from increased glomerular permeability causes the excretion of significant quantities of protein.

Discussions of the renal handling of protein logically tend to focus on albumin because it is by far the most abundant plasma protein. There are, of course, many other plasma proteins. Although present in lower levels than albumin, they are smaller and thus more easily filtered. For example, growth hormone (molecular weight, 22,000 Da) is approximately 60% filterable, and the smaller insulin is 100% filterable. The total mass of these filtered hormones is insignificant; however, because even tiny levels in the plasma have important signaling functions in the body, renal filtration becomes an important influence on concentrations in the blood. Relatively large fractions of these smaller plasma proteins are filtered and then degraded in tubular cells. The kidneys are major sites of catabolism of many plasma proteins, including peptide hormones. Decreased rates of degradation occurring in renal disease may result in elevated plasma hormone concentrations.

Very small peptides are catabolized into amino acids or di- and tripeptides within the proximal tubular lumen by peptidases located on the apical surface of the plasma membrane. These products are then reabsorbed by the same transporters that normally reabsorb filtered amino acids.

Finally, in certain types of renal damage, proteins released from damaged tubular cells may appear in the urine and provide important diagnostic information.

PROXIMAL SECRETION OF ORGANIC SOLUTES

So far we have described reabsorption of useful organic substances the body does not normally excrete. There are of course many organic solutes that it does excrete, both endogenously produced organics and foreign chemicals (see Table 5–1 for a partial listing). This includes most of the solutes in the category of uremic toxins that must be excreted to maintain health. Many of these organics are extensively bound to plasma proteins and undergo glomerular filtration only to a limited extent; accordingly, proximal tubular secretion constitutes the only significant mechanism for their excretion.

Organic Cations

The proximal tubules possess several closely related transport systems for organic cations. Because there are a number of different transporters that are relatively nonselective as to which solute species they accept, a substantial number of foreign and endogenous organic cation species are transported. Although the transporters manifest T_m limitation, in many cases over 90% of a given cation species entering the renal circulation is removed, indicating that the transport capacity is high. The process begins with the Na-K-ATPase, which establishes a potassium concentration gradient and resulting negative membrane potential. Organic cations enter across the basolateral membrane via one of several uniporters, members of the OCT family (Organic Cation Transporter) driven energetically by the negative

Table 5–1. Some organic cations actively secreted by the proximal tubule

Endogenous substances	Drugs
Acetylcholine	Atropine
Choline	Isoproterenol
Creatinine	Cimetidine
Dopamine	Meperidine
Epinephrine	Morphine
Guanidine	Procaine
Histamine	Quinine
Serotonin	Tetraethyl ammonium
Norepinephrine	
Thiamine	

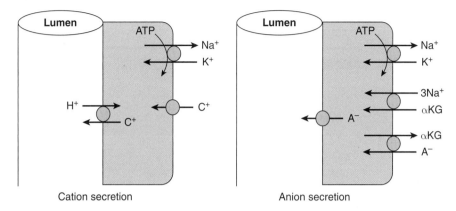

Figure 5–2. Common tubular secretory mechanisms for organic cations and anions. Secreted cations are taken up by the tubular epithelium via OCTs, driven by the negative membrane potential and secreted across the apical membrane via antiporters in exchange for protons. Secreted anions are taken up across the basolateral membrane by antiporters in exchange for αKG. They are secreted across the apical membrane by several different transporters including the multidrug resistant protein MPR-2.

membrane potential. This raises the cytosolic concentration of the cation well above that in the interstitium. The cations then exit into the lumen via an antiporter that exchanges a proton for the organic cation (Figure 5–2). Because this antiporter exchanges two univalent cations, it is electroneutral and unaffected by the membrane potential.

Organic Anions

The active secretory pathway for many organic anions in the proximal tubule uses the recycling of α-ketoglutarate (αKG) as a tool. First, αKG, which is a divalent anion, is actively taken up from both the lumen and interstitium by a sodium-αGK symporter (stoichiometry of three sodium per αKG), which raises the cellular levels of αKG. Then αKG effluxes across the basolateral membrane via an antiporter that imports an organic anion that is destined to be secreted. This antiporter is a member of the OAT family (*Organic Anion Transporter*) of membrane proteins. The αKG keeps recycling, entering with sodium and effluxing back to the interstitium in exchange for the other organic solute. Finally, the second organic solute is secreted across the apical membrane via one of several pathways, including the multidrug resistance protein MPR-2, which is an ATPase that drives the efflux of many different organic anions (Figure 5–2).

Analogous to the transporters for cations, the basolateral membrane of proximal convoluted tubule epithelial cells contains several OAT isoforms, each one accepting multiple solutes to be transported. The proximal tubule thus has the capacity to secrete all the organic anions listed in Table 5–2 and many more. These organic anions are not significantly permeable through tight junctions or lipid membranes, and their transport is characterized by a T_{m}. If the plasma

Table 5–2. Some organic anions actively secreted by the proximal tubule

Endogenous substances	Drugs
Bile salts	Acetazolamide
Fatty acids	Chlorothiazide
Hippurates	Ethacrynate
Hydroxybenzoates	Furosemide
Oxalate	Penicillin
Prostaglandins	Probenecid
Urate	Saccharin
	Salicylates
	Sulfonamides

concentration of an organic anion is too high, it will not be efficiently removed from the blood by the kidneys.

Metabolic transformations in the liver are very important, where many foreign (and endogenous) substances are conjugated with either glucuronate or sulfate. The addition of these groups renders the parent molecule far more water soluble. These conjugates are actively transported by the organic-anion secretory pathway.

Uric Acid (Urate)

Uric acid is continuously put into the blood by the metabolic catabolism of purines. It is a weak acid with a pK of 5.75. At a normal blood pH of 7.4 the largest fraction exists in the dissociated form as the univalent anion, urate. Urate provides a fascinating example of the renal handling of organic anions that is particularly important for clinical medicine and is illustrative of renal pathology. Some urate is excreted via the GI tract, but most is excreted by the kidneys. An increase in the plasma concentration of urate can cause gout, by the deposition of sodium urate crystals in joints. Urate is also thought to be involved in some forms of heart disease and renal disease; therefore, its removal from the blood is important. However, instead of excreting all the urate it can, the kidneys reabsorb most of the filtered urate. Actually there is simultaneous secretion and reabsorption in the proximal tubule, with reabsorption normally dominating. Typically about 90% of the filtered load is reabsorbed, and only 10% is excreted. Whether urate is secreted or reabsorbed depends on the degree to which the relevant transporters are expressed in the apical or basolateral membranes. (It is not clear if any one cell simultaneously secretes and reabsorbs, or if some cells secrete and others reabsorb.) Urate is freely filterable. The reabsorptive pathway is primarily via an antiporter (URAT1) located in the apical membrane of proximal tubule cells. URAT1 is a member of OAT transporter family described earlier in the pathway for secretion of organic anions, but its location in the apical membrane means that it functions to reabsorb. URAT1 takes up urate in exchange for a secreted anion that was itself taken up via a sodium-anion symporter. Urate exits across the basolateral membrane via the uniporter GLUT9. (Although GLUT9 is a member of the GLUT family of glucose uniporters, it functions in the kidney as a urate uniporter).

The secretion of urate follows the process described above for the secretion of other organic anions, namely uptake from the interstitium via an OAT transporter in the basolateral membrane and efflux into the tubule via one of several anion transporters. Given these mechanisms of renal urate handling, the reader should be able to deduce the three ways by which altered renal function can lead to decreased urate excretion and hence increased plasma urate, as in gout: (1) decreased filtration of urate secondary to decreased GFR, (2) excessive reabsorption of urate, and (3) diminished secretion of urate.

pH DEPENDENCE OF PASSIVE REABSORPTION OR SECRETION

Many of the organic solutes handled by the kidney are weak acids or bases and exist in both neutral and ionized forms in the range of pH normally found in the urine. The state of ionization affects both the aqueous solubility and membrane permeability of the substance. Many neutral solutes are permeable in lipid bilayers and may be reabsorbed without assistance of a transporter. As water is reabsorbed from the tubule, any substance remaining in the tubule becomes progressively more concentrated. And as described in Chapter 9, the luminal pH may change substantially during flow through the tubules. Therefore both the progressive concentration of organic solutes and change in pH can influence the degree to which they are reabsorbed by passive diffusion through regions of tubule beyond the proximal tubule.

At low pH, weak acids are predominantly in their neutral (acid form), while at high pH they dissociate into an anion and a proton. Consider the case in which the tubular fluid becomes acidified relative to the plasma, which it does on a typical Western diet. For a weak acid in the tubular fluid, acidification converts much of the acid to the neutral form and therefore increases its permeability. This favors diffusion out of the lumen (reabsorption). Highly acidic urine (low pH) tends to increase passive reabsorption of weak acids (and promote less excretion). For weak bases, the pH dependence is just the opposite. At low pH they are protonated cations (trapped in the lumen). As the urine becomes acidified, more is converted to the impermeable charged form and is trapped in the lumen. Less is reabsorbed passively, and more is excreted. These events are depicted in Figure 5–3. In the top part of the figure, tubular acidification converts weak acids to the neutral form, allowing passive reabsorption, and converts weak bases to cations, trapping them in the lumen. In the bottom part of the figure, tubular alkalization keeps weak acids ionized, and thus trapped in the lumen, and keeps weak bases neutral, allowing their passive reabsorption.

Having said this, what difference does it make? Because so many medically useful drugs are weak organic acids and bases, all these factors have important clinical implications. For example, if one wishes to enhance the excretion of a

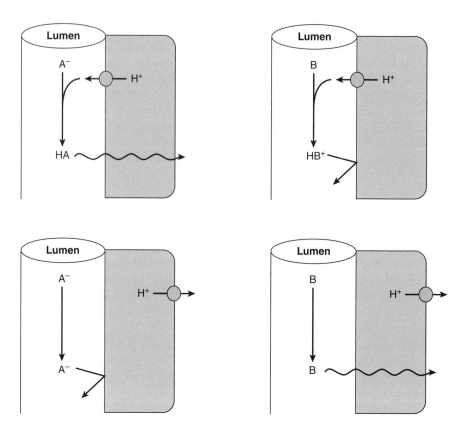

Figure 5–3. Effect of tubular acidification and alkalization of the urine on passive reabsorption of weak acids and bases. Acidification favors reabsorption, and therefore retention, of weak acids because the neutral, protonated forms can passively diffuse out of the tubule (top left). At the same time, acidification favors loss of weak bases because the protonated forms are charged and trapped in the lumen (top right). Alkalization has the opposite effects (bottom left and right). The processes that acidify the urine are described in Chapter 9.

drug that is a weak acid, one attempts to alkalinize the urine (because this traps the ionic form in the lumen). In contrast, acidification of the urine is desirable if one wishes to prevent excretion of the drug. Of course, exactly the opposite applies to weak organic bases. At any luminal fluid pH, increasing the urine flow increases the excretion of both weak acids and bases.

Finally, some organic solutes, although more membrane permeable in the neutral form, are less soluble in aqueous solution and tend to precipitate. This specifically applies to urate. The pK of uric acid is 5.75. In highly acidic urine, increasing fractions of urate exist in the protonated, and less soluble, uric acid form. The combination of excess plasma urate and low urinary pH often leads to uric acid precipitation and the formation of uric acid kidney stones.

UREA

Urea is a very special substance for the kidney. It is an end product of protein metabolism, waste to be excreted, and also an important component for the regulation of water excretion. Urea differs from all the other organic solutes discussed in this chapter in several significant ways. (1) There are no membrane transport mechanisms in the proximal tubule; instead it easily permeates the tight junctions of the proximal tubule so that it is reabsorbed paracellularly. (2) Tubular elements beyond the proximal tubule express urea transporters and handle urea in a complex, regulated manner.

Urea is derived from proteins, which form much of the functional and structural substance of body tissues. Proteins are also a source of metabolic fuel. Dietary protein is first digested into its constituent amino acids. These are then used as building blocks for tissue protein (e.g., muscle), converted to fat or oxidized immediately. During fasting the body breaks down protein into amino acids that are used as fuel, in essence consuming itself. The metabolism of amino acids yields a nitrogen moiety (ammonium) and a carbohydrate moiety. The carbohydrate goes on to further metabolic processing, but the ammonium cannot be further oxidized and is a waste product. Ammonium per se is rather toxic to most tissues (except the medullary interstitium, see Chapter 9) and the liver immediately converts most ammonium to urea and a smaller, but crucial amount to glutamine.

> *Urea constitutes about half the usual solute content of the urine.*

While normal levels of urea are not toxic, the large amounts produced on a daily basis, particularly on a high protein diet, represent a large osmotic load that must be excreted. Whether a person is well-fed or fasting, urea production proceeds continuously and constitutes about half of the usual osmotic content of urine.

The normal level of urea in the blood is quite variable (3–9 mmol/L),[1] reflecting variations in both protein intake and renal handling of urea. Over days to weeks, renal urea excretion must match hepatic production; otherwise, plasma levels would increase into the pathological range (*uremia*). On a shorter term basis (hours to days), urea excretion rate may not exactly match production rate because urea excretion is also regulated for purposes other than keeping a stable plasma level.

The gist of the renal handling of urea is the following: it is freely filtered. About half is reabsorbed passively in the proximal tubule. Then an amount equal to that reabsorbed is secreted back into the loop of Henle, restoring the tubular content to its original value. Finally, about half is reabsorbed a second time in the medullary

---

[1]Plasma urea concentration is usually expressed as blood urea nitrogen (BUN) in units of milligrams per deciliter. Each molecule of urea contains 2 atoms of nitrogen, so 1 mmol of urea contains 2 mmol of nitrogen, with a combined weight of 28 mg. Thus, the normal levels of plasma urea are expressed as BUN values ranging from 8.4 to 25.2 mg/dL. We use units of millimoles per liter because we can then directly convert to osmolality.

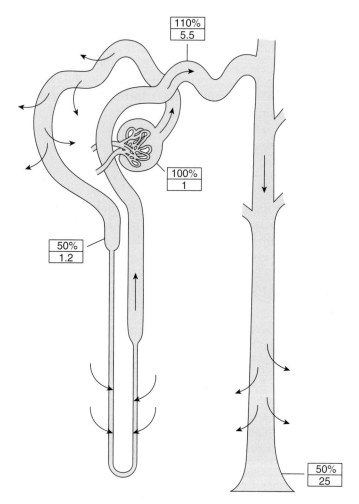

Figure 5–4. Urea handling by the kidney. The arrows indicate that urea is reabsorbed in the proximal tubule, secreted in the thin portions of the loop of Henle, and reabsorbed again in the inner medullary collecting ducts. The top halves of boxes indicate the percentage of the filtered load remaining in the tubule at a given location and the bottom halves indicate tubular concentration relative to plasma. Note that while the amount remaining in the collecting duct (and thus excreted) is half the amount filtered, the *concentration* is much higher than in plasma because most of the water has been reabsorbed. These numbers are highly variable, depending on several factors, particularly the hydration status.

collecting duct. The net result is that about half the filtered load is reabsorbed and half is excreted (Figure 5–4).

As a molecule, urea is small (molecular weight, 60 Da), water soluble, and freely filtered. Because of its highly polar nature, it does not permeate lipid bilayers, but a set of uniporters (UT family) transport urea in various places beyond the proximal tubule and in other sites within the body (particularly red blood cells). Because urea is freely filtered, the filtrate contains urea at a concentration identical to that in plasma. Let us assume a normal plasma level (5 mmol/L). As water is reabsorbed, this concentrates urea to well above 5 mmol/L, and this drives diffusion through the leaky tight junctions. Roughly half the filtered load is reabsorbed in the proximal tubule via the paracellular route. As the tubular fluid enters the loop of Henle, about half the filtered urea remains, but the urea concentration is above its level in the filtrate because proportionally more water than urea was reabsorbed. At this point, the process becomes fairly complicated. First, conditions in the medulla depend highly on the individual's state of hydration. Second, there is a difference between superficial nephrons, with short loops of Henle that only penetrate the outer medulla, and juxtamedullary nephrons, with long loops of Henle that reach all the way down to the papilla. For simplicity we consider all nephrons together.

The interstitium of the medulla has a considerably higher urea concentration than does plasma (for reasons explained later). The concentration increases from the outer to the inner medulla. Since the medullary interstitial urea concentration is greater than that in the tubular fluid entering the loop of Henle, there is a concentration gradient favoring *secretion* into the lumen. The tight junctions in the loop of Henle are no longer permeable (as they were in the cortex), but the epithelial membranes of the *thin* regions of the Henle loops express urea uniporters, members of the UT family. This permits secretion of urea into the tubule. In fact, the urea secreted from the medullary interstitium into the thin regions of the loop of Henle replaces the urea previously reabsorbed in the proximal tubule.

> *Some urea recycles between the tubule and medullary interstitium; about half the filtered load is excreted.*

Thus, when tubular fluid enters the thick ascending limb, the amount of urea in the lumen is at least as large as the filtered load (the loop of Henle has reversed what was accomplished in the proximal tubule). However, because about 80% of the filtered water has now been reabsorbed, the tubular urea *concentration* is now several times greater than in the plasma. Beginning with the *thick* ascending limb and continuing all the way to the inner medullary collecting ducts (through the distal tubule and cortical collecting ducts), the apical membrane urea permeability (and the tight junction permeability) is low. Therefore, an amount of urea roughly equal to the filtered load, but with a considerably higher concentration than in plasma, remains within the tubular lumen and flows from the cortical into the medullary collecting ducts.

During the transit through the cortical collecting ducts variable additional amounts of water are reabsorbed, concentrating the urea even more. Just how much depends on factors discussed in the next chapter, but the luminal urea concentration is well above that of plasma. We indicated earlier that the urea concentration in the medullary interstitium is much greater than in plasma, but the tubular concentration in the medullary collecting ducts is even higher, so in the inner medulla the gradient now favors reabsorption, and urea is reabsorbed a second time, now via another isoform of UT urea uniporter. It is this urea reabsorbed in the inner medulla that leads to the high medullary interstitial concentration driving urea secretion into the thin regions of the loop of Henle. This means that some of the urea *recycles*, that is, it is reabsorbed from inner medullary collecting ducts into the medullary interstitium and secreted into thin limbs of the loop of Henle, from where it travels within the tubule to the collecting ducts again to repeat the process. The overall result of these events is that half the original amount of filtered urea passes into the final urine, an amount that, over the long term, must match hepatic production of urea if the body is to remain in balance for urea. The concentration of urea in the final urine can be more than 50× that in plasma, depending on how much water is reabsorbed. These processes are summarized in Figure 5–4.

KEY CONCEPTS

 Important organic metabolites are reabsorbed almost completely (saved), whereas waste products are for the most part excreted.

 Most organic solutes are transported only in the proximal tubule, usually by a combination of multiporters.

 Normal filtered loads of glucose are completely reabsorbed in the proximal tubule, but in conditions of pathological hyperglycemia the transport saturates, leading to the appearance of glucose in the urine.

 Peptides are reabsorbed either by endocytosis or as individual amino acids following enzymatic degradation on the brush border of the proximal epithelium.

 Some organic solutes, when converted to neutral forms by changes in tubular pH, can be reabsorbed passively in the distal nephron.

 Urea is reabsorbed proximally and recycled between the collecting ducts and loops of Henle in the medulla, resulting in a net excretion of about half the filtered load.

5–1. When plasma glucose reaches such high levels that substantial amounts of glucose appear in the urine (glycosuria):

    a. glucose is leaking back into the tubule through tight junctions.

    b. there is not enough luminal sodium to move in symport with glucose.

    c. all the glucose transporters are working at their maximum rate.

    d. the glucose transporters are being inhibited by the high levels of glucose.

5–2. Useful small organic metabolites that should not be excreted are:

    a. generally not filtered.

    b. reabsorbed paracellularly.

    c. taken up by endocytosis and degraded.

    d. reabsorbed transcellularly.

5–3. Organic anion secretion:

    a. involves a step of active influx across the basolateral membrane.

    b. is passive and paracellular.

    c. occurs via simple diffusion through the tubular membranes.

    d. utilizes the same nonspecific transporters as organic cation secretion.

5–4. A high urinary pH favors:

    a. low excretion of drugs that are weak acids.

    b. active reabsorption of drugs that are weak bases.

    c. low excretion of drugs that are weak bases.

    d. high passive permeability of drugs that are weak acids.

5–5. The tubular concentration of urea

    a. exceeds the plasma concentration at the hairpin turn of the loop of Henle.

    b. decreases to below the plasma concentration by the end of the loop of Henle.

    c. decreases to below the plasma concentration by the end of the proximal tubule.

    d. reaches its highest value in the cortical collecting duct.

5–6. Urea is secreted into the tubules

    a. in proximal tubules.

    b. in the thin descending limbs.

    c. in medullary collecting ducts.

    d. at any of these sites depending on hydration status.

Basic Renal Processes for Sodium, Chloride, and Water

6

OBJECTIVES

- ▶ List approximate percentages of sodium reabsorbed in major tubular segments.
- ▶ List approximate percentages of water reabsorbed in major tubular segments.
- ▶ Describe proximal tubule sodium reabsorption, including the functions of the apical membrane sodium entry mechanisms and the basolateral Na-K-ATPase.
- ▶ Explain why chloride reabsorption is coupled with sodium reabsorption, and list the major pathways of proximal tubule chloride reabsorption.
- ▶ State the maximum and minimum values of urine osmolality.
- ▶ Define osmotic diuresis and water diuresis.
- ▶ Explain why there is always an obligatory water loss.
- ▶ Describe the handling of sodium by the descending and ascending limbs, distal tubule, and collecting-duct system.
- ▶ Describe the role of sodium-potassium-2 chloride symporters in the thick ascending limb.
- ▶ Describe the handling of water by descending and ascending limbs, distal tubule, and collecting-duct system.
- ▶ Describe the process of "separating salt from water" and why this is required to excrete either concentrated or dilute urine.
- ▶ Describe how antidiuretic hormone affects water and urea reabsorption.
- ▶ Describe the characteristics of the medullary osmotic gradient.
- ▶ Explain the role of the thick ascending limb, urea recycling, and medullary blood flow in generating the medullary osmotic gradient.
- ▶ State why the medullary osmotic gradient is partially "washed out" during a water diuresis.

OVERVIEW

This and Chapter 7 are devoted entirely to the renal handling of sodium, chloride, and water. We cover them as a group because their amounts in the body and transport in the kidney are interrelated. First, water constitutes the major fraction of the body volume, specifically including the blood volume, which makes it, in one sense, the most important of all the substances handled by the kidneys. Second, sodium and chloride together account for most of the osmotic content of the extracellular fluid, and therefore its osmolality. Third, the movements of sodium and chloride are mechanistically linked because electroneutrality requires that the movement of sodium, a cation, must be accompanied by the equivalent movement of an anion. As described in Chapter 7, these substances play a huge role in the function of the cardiovascular system and are subject to important, but sometimes rather involved, regulation.

Body Fluid Compartments

 About 60% of the body weight is made up of water, which is distributed into various aqueous spaces in proportion to their osmotic content. The collective volume of all the cells in the body is called the *intracellular fluid* (ICF). It contains roughly two-thirds of the body osmotic content, and therefore two-thirds of the water. The remaining one-third of the osmotic content and water is called the *extracellular fluid* (ECF). It is mostly interstitial fluid (about three-fourth of the ECF) and blood plasma (about one-fourth of the ECF). Because of the ease with which water crosses most cell membranes (see Chapter 4), the ECF and ICF are in osmotic equilibrium. The total of the two volumes varies with gain and loss of water, while the relative proportion of volume in each compartment is influenced by gain and loss of sodium and other solutes. Additions or losses of sodium from the body are mostly to or from the ECF because the actions of cellular Na-K-ATPases prevent major changes in intracellular sodium concentration.[1] If the addition or loss of fluid is isotonic sodium chloride, only the volume of the ECF is affected, but if the fluid is either hyper- or hypo-osmotic, both compartments change volume. These events are depicted in Figure 6–1. The addition of water alone expands both the ICF and ECF (indicated by the dashed lines). Adding sodium chloride without water does not change the total volume, but causes a shift of water from the ICF to the ECF in order to restore equality of osmolality between the two compartments.

> *Volume is distributed between fluid compartments in proportion to their osmotic content.*

Transport of Sodium, Chloride, and Water

The inputs, and therefore excretory rates, of sodium, chloride, and water vary over an extremely wide range. For example, some persons may ingest over 15 g of sodium chloride/day, whereas a person on a low-salt diet may ingest less than 1 g. The normal kidney can readily alter its excretion of salt over this range. Similarly, urinary water excretion can be varied from approximately 0.4 L/day to 25 L/day, depending on whether one is lost in the desert or drinking excessive water for

---

[1]Besides the sodium dissolved in the body fluids there is a considerable amount of sodium in the mineral component of bone that is not osmotically active. In addition, the polysaccharides of connective tissue loosely bind sodium in non-osmotic form.

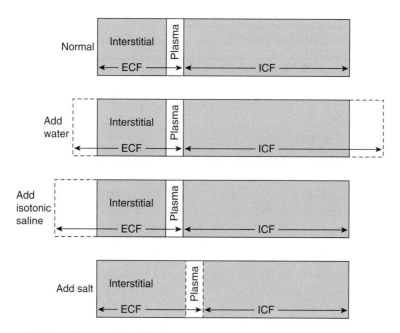

Figure 6-1. Distribution of total body water into the intracellular (ICF) and extracellular (ECF) compartments. Addition of water expands both compartments. Addition of isotonic saline expands only the ECF, while addition of salt without water expands the ECF at the expense of the ICF.

nonphysiological reasons. We know that water and salt are all freely filterable at the renal corpuscle. They all undergo considerable tubular reabsorption (usually more than 99%!), but normally no tubular secretion. Most of the renal ATP energy expended every day is used to accomplish this enormous reabsorptive task. In terms of transport mechanisms, the transport of water is the simplest: it is always reabsorbed; never secreted. And it always moves from a region of lower to higher osmolality (even if the osmotic gradient is very small). As we pointed out in Chapter 4, "water follows the osmoles"; thus much of the description of water reabsorption really amounts to describing solute reabsorption, taking into account the fact that in some regions of the kidney water cannot easily follow the osmoles because the epithelium has very low water permeability. Transport of chloride involves more steps, but is often passive and, because of the constraints of electroneutrality, tied to the transport of sodium.

Sodium transport is admittedly complicated. First, its transport is linked to the transport of many other substances, and second, its rates of transport at various locations along the tubule are subject to regulation

> *Roughly two-thirds of the filtered sodium, chloride, and water are reabsorbed in the proximal tubule in all conditions.*

by multiple controls. However, if we keep in mind the generalized model of epithelial transport developed in Chapter 4 (Figure 4–4) it is not difficult to grasp the key features of sodium transport.

Sodium Reabsorption

Table 6–1 is a balance sheet for sodium. Clearly the major route of sodium excretion from the body under normal circumstances is via the kidneys. The large amount that can be excreted in response to high sodium intake should not obscure the fact that nearly all the filtered sodium is reabsorbed. Table 6–2 summarizes the approximate quantitative contribution of each tubular segment to sodium reabsorption. In an individual with an average salt intake, the proximal tubule reabsorbs 65% of the filtered sodium, the thin and thick ascending limbs of Henle's loop 25%, and the distal convoluted tubule and collecting-duct system most of the remaining 10%, so that the final urine contains less than 1% of the total filtered sodium. As discussed in Chapter 7, reabsorption at several of these tubular sites is under physiological control by multiple signals, so that the exact amount of sodium excreted is homeostatically regulated. Because so much sodium is filtered, even a small percentage change in reabsorption results in a relatively large change in excretion.

Table 6–1. Normal routes and amounts of sodium intake and loss

Route	Amount (g/day)
Intake	
Food	10.5
Output	
Sweat	0.25
Feces	0.25
Urine	10.00
Total output	10.50

Table 6–2. Comparison of sodium and water reabsorption along the tubule

	Percent of filtered load reabsorbed (%)	
Tubular segment	Sodium	Water
Proximal tubule	65	65
Descending thin limb of Henle's loop	—	10
Thin ascending limb and thick ascending limb of Henle's loop	25	—
Distal convoluted tubule	5	—
Collecting-duct system	4–5	5 (during water-loading) >24 (during dehydration)

In all nephron segments, the essential event for active transcellular sodium reabsorption is the primary active transport of sodium from cell to interstitial fluid by the Na-K-ATPase pumps in the basolateral membrane. These pumps keep the intracellular sodium concentration lower than in the surrounding media. Because the inside of the cell is negatively charged with respect to the lumen, there is a large driving force for luminal sodium ions to enter the cell passively either via channels or in symport or antiport with other substances.

Chloride Reabsorption

The tubular locations that reabsorb chloride and the percentages of filtered chloride reabsorbed by these segments are similar to those for sodium because of the constraints of electroneutrality (see Table 6–1). Any volume of fluid *must* contain equal amounts of anion and cation equivalents. One liter of normal filtrate contains 140 mEq of sodium and about 140 mEq of anions, mainly chloride (110 mEq) and bicarbonate (24 mEq). (We say "about" because there are other cations [e.g., potassium and calcium] and anions [e.g., sulfate and phosphate], but their contributions are much smaller than sodium, chloride, and bicarbonate.) If 65% of the sodium in 1 L of filtrate is reabsorbed in the proximal tubule ($0.65 \times 140 = 91$ mEq), then electroneutrality requires that 91 mEq of some combination of chloride and bicarbonate must also be reabsorbed in the proximal tubule to accompany this sodium. As described in Chapter 9, about 90% of the filtered bicarbonate is reabsorbed in the proximal tubule ($0.9 \times 24 \approx 22$). This leaves $91 - 22 = 69$ mEq of chloride that must be reabsorbed in the proximal tubule. This is more than 60% of the filtered chloride and very similar to the fractional reabsorption of sodium. Later segments reabsorb almost all of the remaining 40%.

In active transcellular chloride reabsorption, the critical transport step for chloride is from lumen to cell. The chloride transport process in the luminal membrane must go against the negative membrane potential that repels anions, and it must achieve a high enough intracellular chloride concentration to drive downhill chloride movement out of the cell across the basolateral membrane. Thus, luminal membrane chloride transporters serve essentially the same function for chloride that the basolateral membrane Na-K-ATPase pumps do for sodium: they use energy to move chloride against its electrochemical gradient.

Water Reabsorption

A balance sheet for total body water is given in Table 6–3. These are average values, which are subject to considerable variation. The two sources of body water are metabolically produced water, resulting largely from the oxidation of carbohydrates, and ingested water, obtained from liquids and so-called solid food (e.g., a rare steak is approximately 70% water). There are several sites from which water is always lost to the external environment: skin, lungs, gastrointestinal tract, and kidneys. Menstrual flow and, in lactating women, breast milk constitute two other sources of water loss in women.

The loss of water by evaporation from the cells of the skin and the lining of respiratory passageways is a continuous process, often referred to as *insensible loss* because people are unaware of its occurrence. Additional water evaporates from the skin during production of sweat. Fecal water loss is normally quite small but can be severe in diarrhea. Gastrointestinal loss can also be large during severe bouts of vomiting. Under conditions of normal hydration, the kidneys are, of course, the main route of water loss.

With ingestion of a large water load, the renal response is to produce a large volume of very dilute urine (osmolality much lower than in blood plasma). In contrast, during a state of dehydration, the urine volume is low and very concentrated (i.e., the urine osmolality is much greater than in blood plasma). That the urine osmolality is so variable brings us to a crucial aspect of renal function. Terrestrial animals must be able to independently control excretion of salt and water, because their ingestion and loss is not always linked (see Tables 6–1 and 6–3). To excrete water in excess of salt and vice versa (i.e., produce a range of urine osmolalities), the kidneys must be able to separate the reabsorption of solute from the reabsorption of water, that is, to "separate salt from water," a process described below. Water reabsorption parallels salt reabsorption in the proximal tubule (about 65% of both), but differs in the loop of Henle and beyond. Water is reabsorbed in the early part of the loop (descending portions), while sodium is reabsorbed in the ascending part of the loop. Importantly, the fraction of sodium reabsorbed by the loop as a whole is always greater than that of water. Since the water left behind is now deficient in sodium, the loop overall performs the function of "separating salt from water." When tubular fluid leaves the loop of Henle and enters the distal tubule, the loss of sodium has typically decreased the osmolality to only one-third of the plasma value. In the distal convoluted tubule sodium is reabsorbed, but little or no water, while both occur in the collecting-duct system at highly variable rates depending on body conditions. The complexities just described will make more intuitive sense when seen in the context of specific hydration conditions later on.

Table 6–3. Normal routes of water gain and loss in adults

Route	mL/day
Intake	
Beverage	1200
Food	1000
Metabolically produced	350
Total	2550
Output	
Insensible loss (skin and lungs)	900
Sweat	50
In feces	100
Urine	1500
Total	2550

The majority of water reabsorption occurs through aquaporins in plasma membranes of the tubular cells, and in the proximal tubule through the tight junctions between the cells. The amount of water that moves for a given osmotic gradient and its route depends on the water permeability of the different cellular components. The basolateral membranes of all renal cells are quite permeable to water due to the presence of aquaporins. As a result the cytosolic osmolality is always close to that of the surrounding interstitium. It is the *luminal* membrane and *tight junctions* where most of the variability lies. Only in the proximal tubule are the tight junctions significantly permeable to water. The luminal membranes of the proximal tubule cells are also highly permeable to water as are the luminal membranes of the early parts of the descending thin limb of Henle's loop. In contrast, the luminal membrane of the ascending limbs of Henle's loop and the luminal membranes of distal convoluted tubule are always relatively water *impermeable,* as are the tight junctions. Finally, the water permeability of the luminal membrane of the collecting-duct system is intrinsically low but can be regulated so that its water permeability increases substantially.

The ability of the kidneys to produce low-volume hyperosmotic urine is a major determinant of one's ability to survive without water, which for most people is several days, and even longer under optimal conditions. The human kidney can produce a maximal urinary concentration of 1400 mOsm/kg in extreme dehydration. This is almost five times the osmolality of plasma. The sum of the urea, sulfate, phosphate, other waste products, and a small number of nonwaste ions excreted each day normally averages approximately 600 mOsm/day. Therefore, the minimum volume of water in which this mass of solute can be dissolved is roughly 600 mmol/1400 mOsm/L = 0.43 L/day.

> The continuous excretion of organic waste obligates the loss of water.

This volume of urine is known as the *obligatory water loss.* It is not a strictly fixed value but changes with different physiological states. For example, increased tissue catabolism, as during fasting or trauma, releases excess solute and so increases obligatory water loss.

The obligatory water loss contributes to dehydration when a person is deprived of water and limits survival time. For example, if we could produce urine with an osmolarity of 6000 mOsm/L, the obligatory water loss would only be 100 mL of water, and survival time would be greatly increased. A desert rodent, the kangaroo rat, does just that. This animal does not need to drink water because the water content of its food and the water produced by metabolism of the foods are sufficient to meet its needs.[2]

---

[2]The obligatory solute excretion explains why a thirsty sailor cannot drink sea water, even if the urine osmolality is slightly greater than that of the sea water. To excrete all the salt in 1 L of sea water (to prevent a net gain of salt) plus the obligatory organic solutes produced by the body, the volume of urine would have to be much greater than 1 L.

INDIVIDUAL TUBULAR SEGMENTS
Proximal Tubule

As shown in Figure 6–2, sodium is removed from the tubular lumen and enters proximal tubule cells by several entry steps, the main one in the early portion being antiport with protons from within the cells. Given the large amount of sodium reabsorbed compared with the vanishingly low levels of cellular protons, it might seem that there are not enough protons to supply the transporter. Furthermore something must happen to all those protons once in the lumen. These issues will be described thoroughly in Chapter 9, but for now we note that there is effectively an infinite supply of protons to be secreted because their removal from the cell by antiport results in immediate replacement when carbon dioxide combines with water, a process that produces protons and bicarbonate. The protons are secreted across the luminal membrane in exchange for sodium entry, while bicarbonate exits the cell across the basolateral membrane in symport with

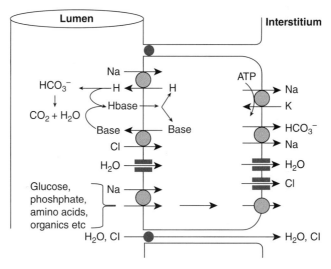

Figure 6–2. Major pathways for reabsorption of sodium, chloride, and water in the proximal tubule. The entire proximal tubule is the major site for reabsorption of salt and water. Sodium entry is coupled to the secretion or uptake of a variety of substances, the major one being secreted hydrogen ions via the NHE-3 antiporter. These hydrogen ions combine with filtered bicarbonate and secreted organic base (see text and Chapter 9 for further explanation). Additional sodium enters in symport with glucose, amino acids, and phosphate. Sodium is transported to the interstitium mostly via the basolateral Na-K-ATPase, but also in symport with bicarbonate. (The coupling between sodium and bicarbonate is described fully in Chapter 9.) Chloride that enters in antiport with organic base leaves mostly via channels. In addition, a substantial amount of chloride is reabsorbed paracellularly. Water moves both paracellularly and intracellularly via aquaporins. ATP, adenosine triphosphate.

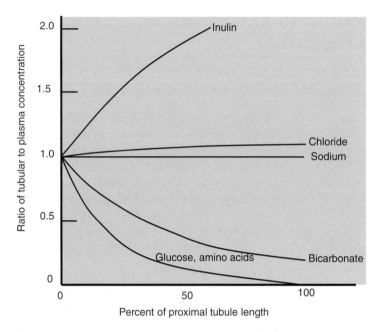

Figure 6–3. Concentrations of selected solutes in tubular fluid relative to concentrations in plasma as a function of distance along proximal tubule. The handling of solutes falls into three rough classes. For substances that are not reabsorbed, such as inulin, the concentration rises markedly due to water reabsorption, thereby concentrating the solute. Sodium and chloride concentrations do not change very much because these solutes and water are reabsorbed in equal roughly proportions. The concentration of bicarbonate progressively falls because it is reabsorbed in greater proportion than water, while the concentrations of useful organic solutes approach zero because they are reabsorbed nearly completely. (Adapted with permission from Rector FC Jr: Sodium, bicarbonate, and chloride absorption by the proximal tubule, *Am J Physiol.* May;244(5):F461-F471.)

sodium. Many of the secreted protons combine with filtered bicarbonate to form carbon dioxide and water once again. Therefore, in the early proximal tubule, bicarbonate is a major anion reabsorbed with sodium, and the luminal bicarbonate concentration decreases markedly (Figure 6–3). The other secreted protons combine with other secreted bases as described below. Organic nutrients such as glucose are also absorbed with sodium, and their luminal concentrations decrease rapidly.

A major percentage of chloride reabsorption in the proximal tubule occurs via paracellular diffusion. Along the early proximal tubule, the reabsorption of water causes the chloride concentration in the tubular lumen to increase somewhat above that in the peritubular capillaries (see Figure 6–4). Then, as the fluid flows through the middle and late proximal tubule, this concentration gradient, maintained by continued water reabsorption, provides the driving force for paracellular chloride reabsorption by diffusion.

There is also an important component of active chloride transport from lumen to cell in the later proximal tubule. As illustrated in Figure 6–3, it uses parallel

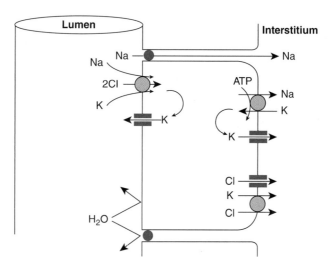

Figure 6–4. Major transport pathways for sodium and chloride in thick ascending limb of the loop of Henle. The key transporter in the thick ascending limb is the Na-K-2Cl symporter (NKCC), which is the target for inhibition by loop diuretics like furosemide and bumetanide. The cells contain potassium channels that recycle potassium from the cell interior to the lumen and to the interstitium (see Chapter 8). Besides transcellular routes, considerable sodium moves paracellularly in response to the lumen-positive potential. The apical membranes and tight junctions have a very low water permeability. Because the cells reabsorb salt, but not water, the thick ascending limb is the region of the nephron in which salt is separated from water. This ultimately allows water excretion and salt excretion to be controlled independently. Defects in NKCC, the recycling potassium channel, and the basolateral chloride channel lead, respectively, to the three different types of Bartter's syndrome. ATP, adenosine triphosphate.

Na-H and Cl-base antiporters. Chloride moves into the cell in exchange for the downhill efflux of organic bases, particularly formate and oxalate. In turn, these bases are driven back into the cell by symport with sodium or protons, which raises their levels within the cell above electrochemical equilibrium, thereby supplying the energy to drive their efflux when they exchange for chloride. Notice that these organic bases endlessly *recycle*, moving into the cells via symport with sodium or protons and then move back out via exchange for chloride. Similarly, protons also recycle, exiting the cells via the NHE antiporter and entering again in symport with a base. The overall achievement of the parallel Na-H and Cl-base antiporters is the same as though the chloride and sodium were simply cotransported into the cell together. Importantly, the recycling of protons and base means that most of the protons are not accumulating in the lumen but are simply combining with the base and moving back into the cells. Finally, chloride leaves the cells across the basolateral membrane via Cl channels and K-Cl symporters. It should also be recognized that everything is ultimately dependent on the basolateral membrane Na-K-ATPases to establish the gradient for sodium that powers the luminal Na-H antiporter and Na-base symporter (Table 6–4).

Table 6–4. Summary of mechanisms by which reabsorption of sodium drives reabsorption of other substances in the proximal tubule

1. Creates transtubular osmolality difference, which favors reabsorption of water by osmosis; in turn, water reabsorption concentrates many luminal solutes (e.g., chloride and urea), thereby favoring their reabsorption by diffusion.
2. Achieves reabsorption of many organic nutrients, phosphate, and sulfate by symport across the luminal membrane.
3. Achieves reabsorption of bicarbonate by secretion of hydrogen ions by antiport across the luminal membrane. These hydrogen ions convert filtered bicarbonate to CO_2 and water, while bicarbonate generated within the cell is transported into the interstitium as described in Chapter 9.
4. Achieves reabsorption of chloride by parallel Na-H and Cl-base antiporters.

The proximal tubule has a very high permeability to water and very small differences in osmolality (less than 1 mOsm/kg H_2O) suffice to drive the reabsorption of water, which parallels solute reabsorption. The osmolality of the freshly filtered tubular fluid at the very beginning of the proximal tubule is, of course, essentially the same as that of plasma and interstitial fluid. As solute is reabsorbed from the proximal tubule the luminal osmolality falls slightly. Simultaneously the reabsorbed solute raises the interstitial fluid osmolality, but not significantly because the high perfusion through peritubular capillaries keeps the interstitial osmolality close to the plasma value. The osmotic gradient from lumen to interstitial fluid, although small, is enough to drive osmosis of water from the lumen across the plasma membranes via aquaporins and tight junctions into the interstitial fluid. The Starling forces across the peritubular capillaries in the interstitium favor reabsorption, as explained in Chapter 4, and so the water and solutes then move into the peritubular capillaries and are returned to the general circulation.

The Loop of Henle

Henle's loop as a whole reabsorbs proportionally more sodium and chloride (about 25% of the filtered loads) than water (10% of the filtered water). The result is that the sodium concentration in the tubular is reduced to the range of ~50 mEq/L and the fluid delivered to the distal nephron (distal tubule and beyond) is hypo-osmotic relative to plasma.

As shown in Table 6–2, the reabsorption of sodium chloride and reabsorption of water occur in different places. The descending limbs reabsorb water, but little or no sodium or chloride. Until just before the hairpin turn the luminal membranes express aquaporins, which allow water to move easily into the cells. The remaining portions of Henle's loop do not express luminal aquaporins and have very low water permeability. The majority of nephrons are superficial nephrons and extend only to the border between the outer and inner medulla before turning. There are fewer long-looped nephrons with thin limbs extending past the border into the inner medulla. Because of this anatomical feature, the vast majority of the water reabsorbed by the loop of Henle occurs in the outer medulla only.

The *ascending* limbs (both thin and thick) reabsorb sodium and chloride but very little water. Fluid entering the ascending limbs has a somewhat elevated sodium and chloride concentration because water was removed in the descending limbs. The thin ascending limb cells express chloride channels in both luminal and basolateral membranes through which passive chloride reabsorption occurs. The tight junctions are somewhat leaky to sodium, and so sodium follows the chloride.

As tubular fluid enters the *thick* ascending limb (at the junction between inner and outer medulla), the transport properties of the epithelium change again, and active processes become dominant. And because most nephrons are short-looped and do not have thin ascending limbs, the vast majority of sodium and chloride reabsorbed by the loop of Henle occurs in the thick ascending limbs in the outer medulla (and of course in the cortex, because all thick ascending limbs continue until they reach their parent Bowman's capsules).

> *The Na-K-2Cl symporter in the thick ascending limb is the machine that separates salt from water.*

As shown in Figure 6–5, the major luminal entry step for the sodium and chloride in thick ascending limbs is via the Na-K-2Cl symporter. This symporter is the target for a major class of diuretics collectively known as the *loop diuretics*,

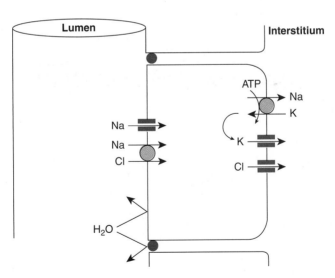

Figure 6–5. Major transport pathways for sodium and chloride in the distal convoluted tubule. The apical membrane contains the Na-Cl symporter (NCC), which is the target for inhibition by thiazide diuretics. There is also some sodium reabsorption via apical sodium channels (ENaCs). The apical membranes and tight junctions have a very low water permeability. A defect in NCC leads to Gitelman's syndrome. ATP, adenosine triphosphate.

which include the drugs furosemide (Lasix) and bumetanide. The stoichiometry of the Na-K-2Cl symporter has several important consequences. First, it requires that equal amounts of potassium and sodium be transported into the cell. There is far less potassium in the lumen than sodium, but the luminal membrane has a large number of potassium channels that allow much of the potassium to leak back, that is, potassium recycles between the cytosol and lumen. Thus, under normal circumstances, luminal potassium does not limit sodium and chloride reabsorption through Na-K-2Cl symporters.

The Na-K-2Cl symporter moves twice as much chloride as sodium into the cell, therefore twice as much chloride must also exit the cell across the basolateral membrane, creating what at first glance might seem to be a violation of electro-neutrality. The chloride leaves by a combination of chloride channels and chloride-potassium symporters, while sodium leaves primarily via the Na-K-ATPase. Since two chloride ions enter the cell for every two cations (one sodium and one potassium), and potassium tends to recycle back across the apical membrane, there has to be another pathway for sodium to balance the flux of chloride. This pathway is the paracellular route through tight junctions. The movement of chloride sets up a lumen-positive potential that drives sodium (and other cations) paracellularly. Thus, about half the sodium moves through the cells and half moves by paracellular diffusion. There is also some entrance of sodium via apical Na-H antiporters that are responsible for reabsorption of most of the remaining tubular bicarbonate. Of course, none of these transcellular or paracellular mechanisms would work without the continuous operation of the Na-K-ATPase in the basolateral membrane.

To summarize the most important features of the loop of Henle, the descending limb reabsorbs water but little sodium chloride, mostly in the outer medulla. The ascending limb reabsorbs sodium chloride but little water, mostly in the outer medulla and cortex. The net of the loop as a whole is reabsorption of more salt than water. The ascending limb is called a *diluting segment*, because the fluid leaving the loop to enter the distal convoluted tubule is hypo-osmotic (more dilute) compared with plasma.

Distal Convoluted Tubule

First, let us clarify some admittedly confusing terminology. Tubular elements beyond the loop of Henle include the distal convoluted tubule, connecting tubule, and cortical collecting duct, all of which exist only in the cortex. These are followed by the outer medullary collecting duct and inner medullary collecting ducts. These elements together are often called the "distal nephron." Cells of the late distal tubule and beyond are regulated in part by the hormone aldosterone, as described in Chapter 7, and are called the "aldosterone-sensitive distal nephron." The distal tubule itself lies entirely within the cortex, beginning just after the macula densa where the tubule passes between the afferent and efferent arterioles at the vascular pole of the Bowman's capsule. It parallels the activity of the thick ascending limb by reabsorbing salt with little water, and therefore is also a diluting segment, although it uses different transport mechanisms. The major luminal entry step in the active reabsorption of sodium and chloride by the early part

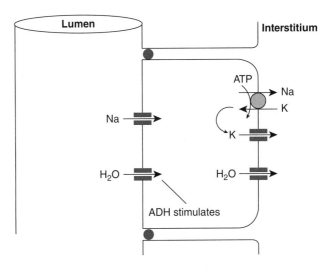

Figure 6–6. Major transport pathways for sodium, chloride, and water in principal cells of the cortical collecting duct, which are the major cell type. Sodium reabsorption is via apical sodium channels (ENaC). Chloride reabsorption is mainly transcellular via intercalated cells (see Chapter 9). Water reabsorption is via aquaporins, the activity of which is controlled by the antidiuretic hormone (ADH). ATP, adenosine triphosphate.

of the distal convoluted tubule is via the Na-Cl symporter (Figure 6–6). The characteristics of this transporter differ significantly from the Na-K-2Cl symporter. It is sensitive to different drugs. In particular, the Na-Cl symporter is blocked by the thiazide diuretics including hydrochlorothiazide and chlorthalidone, which makes it a major site for pharmacological intervention. Sodium exits the cell by the Na-K-ATPase, while chloride leaves via channels and a K-Cl symporter.

Connecting Tubule and Collecting-Duct System

In the late distal tubule, there is a gradual transition in cell types from those that reabsorb sodium by Na-Cl symporters to those that take up sodium via sodium channels (ENaC). In addition, the connecting tubule begins an entirely new task—it reabsorbs water in highly variable amounts that depend on body conditions. Furthermore cells of the connecting tubule and beyond have major mechanisms to control potassium and acid/base excretion, as described in later chapters.

> *Most filtered water is reabsorbed proximally. Variable amounts of what remains are reabsorbed distally under the control of ADH.*

The tubular epithelium in the connecting tubule and beyond is characterized by principal cells (so-called because they make up approximately 70% of the cells; Figure 6–7) and at least three types of intercalated cells, that is, cells

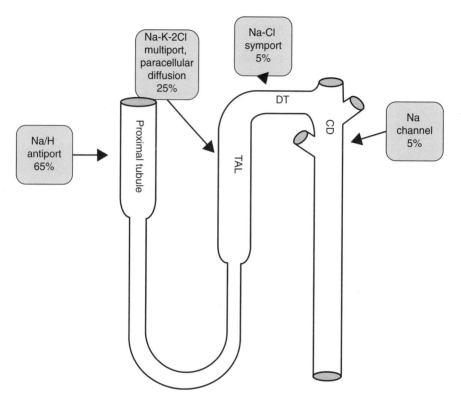

Figure 6–7. Major mechanisms for sodium reabsorption along the tubule, with the percentage of filtered load reabsorbed at the indicated locations.

that are intercalated between the principal cells. Reabsorption of both sodium and water occurs in principal cells. As these cells reabsorb sodium, the luminal entry step is via epithelial sodium channels (ENaC). Regulation of this entry step is enormously important for whole-body physiology, and we expand on this topic in Chapter 7.

The handling of chloride in the distal nephron is rather complex because the handling of solutes other than sodium makes up a significant component of ion transport. Chloride moves in an interplay between several types of intercalated cells that are key players in potassium and acid-base transport described in Chapters 8 and 9 (see Figure 9–3). As in all nephron segments, however, net anion flux must equal net cation flux. Thus chloride flux must match the net of sodium, potassium, and acid-base transport.

How does the collecting-duct system handle water? As tubular fluid enters the collecting-duct system in the cortex the luminal osmolality is low, typically a little above 100 mOsm/kg. The tubules at this point are surrounded by the cortical interstitium having the same osmolality as plasma (285 mOsm/kg). Therefore there is a large osmotic gradient favoring water reabsorption. The amount of water reabsorbed varies with the tubular water permeability, which is finely regulated in principal cells by circulating antidiuretic hormone (ADH; see Figure 6–8). The inner medullary collecting duct has at least a finite water permeability even in the absence of ADH, but the outer medullary and cortical regions have a very low water permeability without the actions of this hormone.

Consider the case when a person is well-hydrated. There is little ADH; consequently water permeability is very low. The hypo-osmotic fluid entering the collecting-duct system from the distal convoluted tubule remains hypo-osmotic as it flows along the ducts. When this fluid reaches the medullary portion of the collecting ducts there is now a very large osmotic gradient favoring reabsorption. Some water is reabsorbed in the medullary region, but most of the water flows on to the ureter. The result is the excretion of a large volume of very hypo-osmotic (dilute) urine, or *water diuresis*. Recall that almost 25% of the filtered water is still within the tubule at the beginning of the collecting-duct system, so this amounts to a huge amount of nonreabsorbed water.

Even when very little water reabsorption occurs beyond the loop of Henle, the reabsorption of sodium is not reduced to any great extent. Therefore, the tubular sodium concentration can be lowered almost to zero in these segments, and the osmolality can approach 50 mOsm/kg, most of the osmotic content being made up of urea and other organic waste. The low sodium is possible because these tubular segments are "tight" epithelia, and there is very little back-leak of sodium from interstitium to tubular lumen despite the large electrochemical gradient favoring diffusion.

Now consider the situation when the body is conserving water (high ADH). As the hypo-osmotic fluid enters the cortical segments of the collecting-duct system most of the water is rapidly reabsorbed. This is driven by the large difference in osmolality between the hypo-osmotic luminal fluid and the iso-osmotic interstitial fluid of the cortex. In essence, the cortical collecting duct *reverses* the dilution carried out by the diluting segments. Once the osmolality of the luminal fluid approaches that of the interstitial fluid, the cortical collecting duct then behaves analogously to the proximal tubule, reabsorbing approximately equal proportions of solute (mainly sodium chloride) and water. The result is that the tubular fluid entering the medullary collecting duct is greatly reduced in volume and is iso-osmotic with cortical plasma.

In the medullary collecting duct solute reabsorption continues but water reabsorption is proportionally even greater. The tubular fluid becomes further reduced in volume and very hyperosmotic because the interstitial fluid of the medulla is very hyperosmotic (for reasons discussed later). Water handling during the extremes of diuresis and antidiuresis is depicted in Figure 6–8.

Cellular Mechanism of ADH

An alternative name for ADH is vasopressin, because the hormone can constrict arterioles and thus increase arterial blood pressure, but ADH's major renal effect is antidiuresis (i.e., "against a high urine volume"). ADH acts in the collecting ducts on the principal cells, the same cells that reabsorb sodium. The renal receptors for ADH (vasopressin type 2 receptors) are expressed in the basolateral membrane

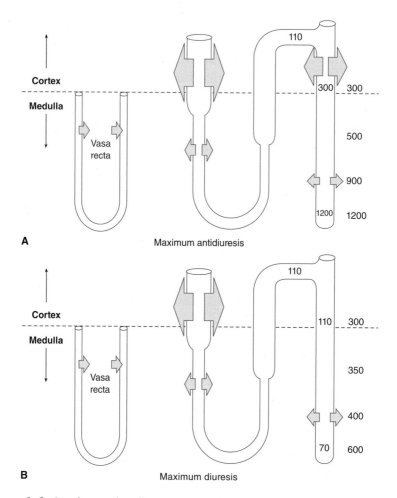

A   Maximum antidiuresis

B   Maximum diuresis

Figure 6–8. Renal water handling in states of maximum antidiuresis and maximum diuresis. Numbers to the right indicate interstitial osmolality; numbers in the tubules indicate luminal osmolality. The dashed line indicates the cortico-medullary border. Arrows indicate sites of water movement. In both antidiuresis and diuresis, most (65%) of the filtered water is reabsorbed in the proximal tubule and another 10% in the descending loop of Henle. The greater relative reabsorption of solute versus water by the loop as a whole and distal tubule results in luminal fluid that is quite dilute (110 mOsm) as it enters the collecting ducts. During antidiuresis (**A**), the actions of antidiuretic hormone permit most remaining water to be reabsorbed in the cortical collecting duct. Additional reabsorption in the medullary collecting results in final fluid that is very hyperosmotic (1200 mOsm). During diuresis (**B**), no water reabsorption occurs in the cortical collecting tubule, but some occurs in the inner medullary collecting tubule independent of ADH. Despite the medullary water reabsorption, continued medullary solute reabsorption reduces solute content relatively more than water content and the final urine is very dilute (70 mOsm). In the parallel vasa recta, there is considerable exchange of both solute and water. The ascending vasa recta ultimately remove all the solute and water reabsorbed in the medulla. Because there is always some net volume reabsorption in the medulla, the vasa recta plasma flow out of the medulla always exceeds the plasma flow in.

of the principal cells and are different from the vascular receptors (vasopressin type 1). The binding of ADH by its receptors results in the activation of adenylate cyclase, which catalyzes the intracellular production of cyclic adenosine monophosphate (cAMP). This second messenger then induces, by a sequence of events, the migration of intracellular vesicles to, and their fusion with, the luminal membrane. Recall from Chapter 4, this is one of ways of regulating membrane permeability. The vesicles contain aquaporin 2, through which water can move, so the luminal membrane becomes highly permeable to water. In the absence of ADH, the aquaporins are withdrawn from the luminal membrane by endocytosis. (As stated earlier, the water permeability of the *basolateral* membranes of renal epithelial cells is always high because of the constitutive presence of other aquaporin isoforms; thus, the permeability of the luminal membrane is rate limiting.)

URINARY CONCENTRATION: THE MEDULLARY OSMOTIC GRADIENT

The production of hyperosmotic urine requires that the tubules pass through a region of hyperosmotic interstitium to provide the osmotic drawing power to concentrate the tubular fluid. The question is, how do the kidneys generate a medullary interstitium that is hyperosmotic relative to plasma? Not only is the medullary interstitium hyperosmotic, but there is a *gradient* of osmolality, increasing from a nearly iso-osmotic value at the corticomedullary border, to a maximum of greater than 1000 mOsm/kg at the papilla. This peak value is not rigidly fixed; it is a variable that changes depending on the state of hydration (or pathologically on urea production). It is highest during periods of water deprivation and dehydration, when urinary excretion is lowest, and is "washed out" to only about half of that during excess hydration and when urinary excretion is high. Some aspects of how the kidneys generate a medullary osmotic gradient are still uncertain. However, the essential points are clear, and it is these essential points on which we now focus.[3]

We should first differentiate between the *development* of the medullary osmotic gradient, as opposed to its maintenance once established. In the steady state there must be mass balance, that is, every substance that enters the medulla via tubule or blood vessel must leave the medulla via tubule or blood vessel. However, during development of the gradient there are transient accumulations of solute, and during washout of the gradient there are losses. In describing the medullary osmotic gradient, it is easiest conceptually to start from a condition in which there is no gradient, and then follow its development over time. The main components of the system that develops the medullary osmotic

---

[3]For simplicity and clarity we have chosen to describe the medullary osmotic gradient without some of the vocabulary found in most texts and discussions, such as "countercurrent multiplier," "single effect," and "passive mechanism." These are terms developed in historical models of the renal medulla that may be supplanted by more recent findings, such as the events in local microenvironments created by the anatomic clustering of tubular and vascular elements.

gradient are (1) active NaCl transport by the thick ascending limb, (2) the very low water permeability of the apical membranes of thick ascending limb cells, (3) the parallel arrangement of blood vessels and tubular segments in the medulla, with descending components in close apposition to ascending components, and (4) the recycling of urea between the medullary collecting ducts and the deep portions of the loops of Henle (Figure 5–4).

> *Without active sodium reabsorption by the thick ascending limb there would be no osmotic gradient.*

The absolute requirement to develop the osmotic gradient in the medullary interstitium is deposition of solute in excess of water. In the outer medulla, this is accomplished by reabsorbing more salt than water, that is, sodium and chloride reabsorbed by the thick ascending limb exceeds the reabsorption of water by the thin descending limbs; the net of the two processes being deposition of hyperosmotic fluid in the outer medulla. At the junction between the inner and outer medulla, the ascending limbs of all loops of Henle, whether long or short, turn into thick regions and remain thick all the way until they reach the original Bowman's capsules from which the tubule originally arose in the cortex. As they reabsorb solute with very little or no water and dilute the luminal fluid, they add this solute without water to the surrounding interstitium. This action of the thick ascending limb is absolutely essential and is the key to everything else that happens. If transport in the thick ascending limb is inhibited (by loop diuretics that block the Na-K-2Cl symporter), the lumen is not diluted and the interstitium is not concentrated, and the urine becomes iso-osmotic. For those portions of the thick ascending limb in the cortex, the reabsorbed solute simply mixes with material reabsorbed by the nearby proximal convoluted tubules. Because the cortex contains abundant peritubular capillaries and a high blood flow, the reabsorbed salt immediately moves into the vasculature and returns to the general circulation. However, in the medulla, the vascular anatomy is arranged differently and total blood flow is much lower. Solute that is reabsorbed and deposited in the outer medullary interstitium during the establishment of the osmotic gradient accumulates. The degree of accumulation before a steady state is reached is a function of the arrangement of the vasa recta, their permeability properties and the volume of blood flowing within them.

> *The medullary osmotic gradient is composed mostly of NaCl in the outer medulla and urea in the inner medulla.*

If there were no blood flow, sodium transported out of the thick ascending limb would accumulate in the outer medulla without limit, because there would be no way to remove it. But of course the outer medulla is perfused with blood as are all tissues. Blood enters and leaves the outer medulla through parallel bundles of descending and ascending vasa recta, connected at their bottom by a capillary plexus (not a hairpin loop).

1. Sodium is reabsorbed from the thick ascending limb into the outer medulla and distributed to the inner medulla via descending vasa recta.
2. Water diffuses from descending to ascending vasa recta (countercurrent exchange).
3. Urea recycles from inner medullary collecting ducts to thin limbs of the loop of Henle.

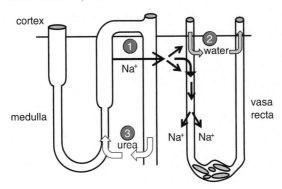

Figure 6–9. Key processes that generate the medullary osmotic gradient. Process 1 is the active transport of sodium from the loop of Henle into the interstitium of the outer medulla and its distribution deeper into the medulla via descending vasa recta (solid arrows). Process 2 is the countercurrent movement of water from descending to ascending vasa recta (filled arrow). Process 3 is the recycling of urea from the inner medullary collecting ducts to the loop of Henle (dashed arrows).

Both the ascending and descending vasa recta as well as the capillaries are permeable to sodium. Therefore sodium enters the vasa recta driven by the rise in concentration in the surrounding interstitium. Sodium entering the ascending vessels returns to the general circulation, but sodium in the descending vessels is distributed deeper into the medulla, where it diffuses out across the endothelia of the vasa recta and the interbundle capillaries, thereby raising the sodium content (and osmolality) throughout the medulla (see Figure 6–9). It is here that the anatomy of the vasculature becomes particularly important. If medullary blood with its somewhat elevated sodium concentration simply flowed into a venous drainage system, there would be no additional increase in sodium concentration. However, the interbundle capillaries drain into ascending vasa recta that lie near descending vasa recta. The walls of the ascending vasa recta are fenestrated, allowing movement of water and small solutes between plasma and interstitium. As the sodium concentration of the medullary interstitium rises, it diffuses into the ascending vessels, which also take on an increasingly higher sodium concentration. However, blood *entering* the medulla always has a normal sodium concentration (about 140 mEq/L). Accordingly, some of the sodium recirculates, diffusing out of ascending vessels and reentering nearby descending vessels that contain less sodium. The process of moving from ascending to descending vessels is called *countercurrent exchange*. Over time everything reaches a steady state in which the amount of new sodium entering the interstitium from thick ascending limbs matches the amount of sodium leaving the interstitium in ascending vasa recta. At its peak, the concentration of sodium in the medulla may reach 300 mEq/L, more than double its value in the general circulation. Since sodium is accompanied by an anion, mostly chloride, the contribution of salt to the medullary osmolality is about 600 mOsm/kg.

Before describing the consequences of the increased levels of sodium in the medullary interstitium, several constraining principles should be kept in mind: (1) While solute can accumulate without a major effect on renal volume, the amount of water in the medullary interstitium must remain nearly constant; otherwise the medulla would undergo significant swelling or shrinking. (2) Because water is always entering the interstitium by reabsorption from descending thin limbs and medullary collecting ducts, that water must be removed by entrance into the vasculature. (3) Blood entering the medulla has passed through glomeruli, thereby concentrating the plasma proteins. While the overall osmotic content (osmolality) of this blood is essentially isosmotic with systemic plasma, its *oncotic* pressure is considerably higher.

The endothelial cells of descending vasa recta contain aquaporins. Water is drawn osmotically from these blood vessels into the outer medullary interstitium by the high salt content in a manner similar to water being drawn out of tubular elements. The loss of water from descending vasa recta serves the useful purpose of raising the osmolality of blood traveling down into the inner medulla and decreasing its volume, thereby reducing the tendency to dilute the inner medullary interstitium. The ascending vasa recta have a fenestrated endothelium, allowing free movement of water and small solutes. Since the oncotic pressure is high, water in the interstitium of the outer medulla is taken up by ascending vasa recta and removed, that is, water crosses from descending to ascending vasa recta. Just as there is countercurrent exchange of solute between descending and ascending vessels, there is countercurrent exchange of water. In descending vessels water leaves and solute enters, while in ascending vessels water enters and solute leaves (see Figures 1–5 and 6–9). It is the countercurrent movement of water that prevents entering blood from diluting the inner medulla because that water never gets there. All water reabsorbed from tubular elements is taken up by capillaries and ascending vasa recta and removed, thereby preserving constancy of total medullary water content.

> *Countercurrent blood flow prevents the immediate removal of reabsorbed solute.*

The *magnitude* of blood flow in the vasa recta is a crucial variable. The peak osmolality in the interstitium depends on the ratio of sodium pumping by the thick ascending limbs to blood flow in the vasa recta. If this ratio is high (meaning low blood flow), water from the isosmotic plasma entering the medulla in descending vasa recta does not dilute the hyperosmotic interstitium. In effect the "salt wins" and osmolality remains at a maximum. But in conditions of water excess, this ratio is lower (high blood flow) and the diluting effect of water diffusing out of descending vasa recta is considerable. In part the tendency to dilute is controlled by ADH. As well as increasing water permeability in the collecting ducts, ADH vasoconstricts the pericytes that surround descending vasa recta, thereby limiting their blood flow. Thus, when water is being conserved (high ADH), medullary blood flow is reduced and the high osmolality is preserved.

The third major player involved in the development of the medullary osmotic gradient is urea. As indicated above, the peak osmolality in the renal papilla reaches over 1000 mOsm/kg. About half of this is accounted for by sodium and chloride, and most of the rest is (500–600 mOsm/kg) is accounted for by urea. To develop such a high concentration of urea (remember that the normal plasma concentration is only about 5 mmol/L) there must be a process of recycling. This involves the tubules as well as the vasa recta.

We described this recycling process in Chapter 5 and review it here. Urea is freely filtered and about half is reabsorbed in the proximal tubule. Urea is secreted in the loop of Henle (thin regions), driven by the high urea concentration in the medullary interstitium. This essentially restores the amount of tubular urea back to the filtered load. From the end of the thin limbs to the inner medullary collecting ducts, little urea transport occurs, so all urea arriving at the thick ascending limb is still there at the start of the inner medullary collecting ducts. Because the vast majority of water has already been reabsorbed prior to the inner medullary collecting ducts (by the cortical and outer medullary collecting ducts), the tubular urea *concentration* has risen up to 50 times its plasma value (i.e., 500 mmol/L or more). In the inner medullary collecting ducts about half the urea is reabsorbed via urea uniporters and the other half is excreted. Because blood flow in this region is so low in conditions of antidiuresis (high ADH), the reabsorbed urea accumulates and raises the interstitial concentration close to that in the lumen. (It is this high interstitial concentration that drives secretion into the thin limbs). The combination of high urea, along with the high sodium and chloride, brings the medullary osmolality to a value exceeding 1000 mOsM/kg. The importance of urea in contributing to the medullary osmotic gradient is emphasized in the case of low protein intake (or starvation), which results in a greatly reduced metabolic production of urea. In this condition, the ability of the kidneys to generate a hyperosmotic medullary interstitium is reduced.

Review of Control by ADH

As emphasized earlier, a key regulator of the osmotic gradient is ADH, which in addition to raising water permeability in the cortical and medullary collecting ducts and constricting pericytes surrounding descending vasa recta also raises urea permeability in the inner medullary collecting ducts by stimulating specific ADH-sensitive isoforms of urea uniporters. Consider how this affects the medullary osmotic gradient. When a person is severely dehydrated, glomerular filtration rate (GFR) is somewhat low and levels of ADH are high. The extraction of water in the cortical collecting duct removes most of the water from the lumen (and makes it iso-osmotic with the cortical interstitium, i.e., about 300 mOsm/kg).

Then, as the remaining but greatly reduced volume flows through the high osmolality medulla, further concentration occurs. The increased urea permeability signaled by ADH greatly assists in generating the medullary osmotic gradient by permitting the medullary concentration and recycling of urea.

Contrast this with a state of overhydration. Some of the medullary solute is washed out and the magnitude of the osmotic gradient is reduced. How does this occur? In states of overhydration levels of ADH are low. GFR is normal, or possibly increased depending on the effectiveness of autoregulation. Most of the tubular fluid entering the cortical collecting ducts flows on through to the medullary collecting ducts. Therefore, tubular urea does *not* become concentrated nearly as much. A high volume of very dilute fluid with a modest urea concentration is delivered to the inner medullary collecting ducts. In contrast to the cortical and outer medullary collecting ducts, which are nearly water impermeable in the absence of ADH, the *inner* medullary collecting ducts have a finite water permeability in the absence of ADH. Although this water permeability is not large, the osmotic driving force is huge, so substantial amounts of water are reabsorbed. (However, even more is *not* reabsorbed, and so the urine volume is still very large.) Not much urea is reabsorbed; in fact, it may be secreted briefly because the luminal urea concentration is lower than in the medullary interstitium. The result of the water reabsorption and the low urea reabsorption is that the inner medulla becomes partially diluted (i.e., the urea concentration and total osmolality of the medullary interstitium decrease over time). The osmolality falls to about half of its value, from well over 1000 mOsm/kg down to 500 to 600 mOsm/kg (Table 6–5). Figure 6–10 depicts renal water fluxes in the two extremes of maximum diuresis and antidiuresis.

To summarize the generation of the renal osmotic gradient (Figure 6–9), salt (without water) is deposited in the interstitium by the thick ascending limb. That

Table 6–5. Composition of medullary interstitial fluid and urine during the formation of a concentrated urine or a dilute urine

Interstitial fluid at tip of medulla (mOsm/L)	Urine (mOsm/L)
	Concentrated urine
Urea = 650	Urea = 700
$Na^+ + Cl^- = 750$*	Nonurea solutes = 700 (Na^+, Cl^-, K^+, urate, creatinine, etc.)
	Dilute urine
Urea = 300	Urea = 30–60
$Na^+ + Cl^- = 350$*	Nonurea solutes = 10–40 (Na^+, Cl^-, K^+, urate, creatinine, etc.)[†]

*Some other ions (e.g., K^+) contribute to a small degree to this osmolarity.

[†]Depending on the sodium balance state, sodium in the urine can vary between undetectable and the majority of the osmolytes.

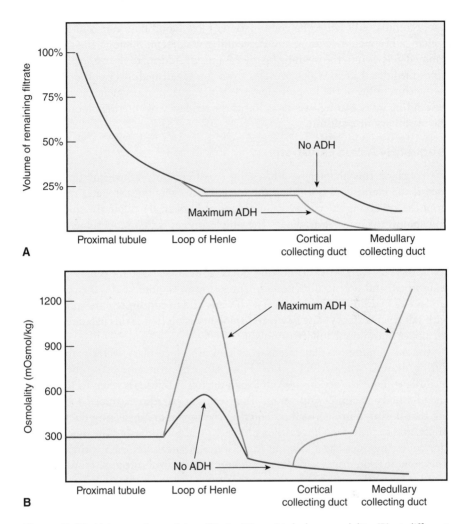

Figure 6–10. Volume of remaining filtrate (**A**) and tubular osmolality (**B**) at different sites along the tubule in conditions of maximum ADH (dashed curves) and no ADH. Under all conditions the majority of the filtered volume is reabsorbed in the proximal tubule. Additional reabsorption occurs in the thin limbs of the loop of Henle, the exact amount depending on ADH because the interstitial osmolality varies with ADH. In the absence of ADH no further reabsorption occurs until the inner medulla, whereas with maximal ADH most of the remaining volume is reabsorbed in the cortical collecting ducts. The osmolality of the final urine is strongly dependent on ADH, as is the maximum osmolality in the loop of Henle because the peak medullary interstitial osmolality also varies with ADH.

salt accumulates because of a combination of low blood flow and countercurrent exchange between ascending and descending vasa recta. Some of the salt is distributed deeper into the medulla by the vasa recta. Adding to the osmolality of the inner medulla is urea, which recycles from the inner medullary collecting ducts to the thin limbs of the loop of Henle. Countercurrent movement of water from descending to ascending vasa recta limits the tendency of entering blood to dilute the medullary interstitium.

Frequently Asked Questions

We conclude this chapter by addressing two frequently asked questions. First, even if the blood does not dilute the interstitium, why doesn't water reabsorbed from the collecting ducts under conditions of high ADH dilute the interstitium and abolish the osmotic gradient? The simple answer is that more solute is deposited into the medulla than water. While some water is reabsorbed from medullary collecting ducts aided by the actions of ADH, most of the water has already been reabsorbed by the cortical collecting ducts, so that the amount remaining to be reabsorbed, and potentially dilute the interstitium, is quite small. The competing tendencies to dilute the interstitium with water and to concentrate the interstitium with salt reach a steady state in which osmolality is high. It is this balance that sets the upper limit on medullary osmolality.

The other question that often arises concerns medullary water reabsorption during diuresis when ADH is low. How can *more* water be reabsorbed in the medulla without the actions of ADH than during antidiuresis when ADH is high and the body is conserving water? This seeming paradox is resolved by realizing that during diuresis the fluid entering the medullary collecting ducts is very dilute, and so provides a huge driving force for reabsorption, and the inner medullary collecting duct has a low, but finite water permeability even without ADH. This combination drives a moderate amount of water reabsorption. However, this amount is greatly exceeded by the amount *not* reabsorbed, that is, excreted.

Figure 6–10 summarizes the previously described changes in volume and osmolality of the tubular fluid as it flows along the nephron and emphasizes how, once fluid enters the collecting-duct system, the osmolality depends very much on levels of ADH.

KEY CONCEPTS

 Most of the body consists of fluid compartments divided into the intracellular fluid (ICF), all the cytosolic volumes collectively, and the extracellular fluid (ECF), consisting mostly of interstitial fluid and blood plasma.

 The reabsorption of most of the filtered water, anions (primarily chloride and bicarbonate), and osmotic content is linked directly to the active reabsorption of sodium.

In all conditions, the vast majority (roughly two-thirds) of the sodium, chloride, bicarbonate, and filtered volume is reabsorbed iso-osmotically in the proximal tubule.

 The loop of Henle reabsorbs some water and proportionally even more sodium, thereby diluting the tubular fluid.

 The distal tubule continues the reabsorption of sodium without water and, along with the loop of Henle, is considered a "diluting segment."

 Reabsorption of water in the distal nephron (connecting tubule and collecting ducts) is highly variable depending on hydration status, allowing the kidneys to excrete large amounts of water or to conserve almost all of it.

 Levels of ADH determine whether the hypo-osmotic fluid entering the distal nephron is excreted largely as is or subsequently reabsorbed.

 The conservation of water and concentration of the urine requires the reabsorption of water into the high osmolality medullary interstitium.

 The medullary osmotic gradient is created by (1) transport of salt with little or no water into the medullary interstitium by the thick ascending limb, (2) low-volume countercurrent blood flow in the vasa recta, and (3) recycling of urea.

 ## STUDY QUESTIONS

6–1. Chloride reabsorption parallels sodium reabsorption mainly because:

a. most chloride transport is via a symporter with sodium.

b. chloride is the most abundant negatively charged species available to balance the reabsorption of the positive charge on sodium.

c. chloride has such a high passive permeability.

d. chloride and sodium are both part of the sodium chloride molecule and cannot be separated.

6–2. The obligatory water loss in the kidney:

a. is another name for insensible loss of water.

b. occurs because there is always at least some excretion of waste solutes.

c. occurs because there is an upper limit to how fast aquaporins can reabsorb water.

d. is the amount of water that accompanies sodium excretion.

6–3.　Which region of the tubule secretes water?

    a.　The descending thin limb.

    b.　The cortical collecting duct.

    c.　The medullary collecting duct (when ADH is absent).

    d.　No region secretes water.

6–4.　If the thick ascending limb stopped reabsorbing sodium, then the final urine would be:

    a.　iso-osmotic with plasma in all conditions.

    b.　dilute.

    c.　concentrated.

    d.　dilute or concentrated, depending on ADH.

6–5.　If a healthy young person drinks a large amount of water, which of the following is unlikely to happen?

    a.　A decrease in osmolality of the cortical interstitium.

    b.　An increase in water permeability in the medullary collecting ducts.

    c.　A decrease in interstitial osmolality in the inner medulla.

    d.　A decrease in the urea concentration in the final urine.

6–6.　A healthy young person drinks a large amount of water. Over the next several hours most of the water filtered by the glomerulus is

    a.　excreted.

    b.　reabsorbed in the proximal tubule.

    c.　reabsorbed in the loop of Henle.

    d.　reabsorbed in the cortical collecting-duct system.

Regulation of Sodium and Water Excretion

7

OBJECTIVES

- Describe how the excretion of salt and water supports the function of the cardiovascular system.
- Name the major regulators of sodium excretion.
- Describe the systemic renin-angiotensin-aldosterone system and where its components are formed.
- State the major actions of angiotensin II.
- State the major actions of aldosterone.
- Describe the three major regulators of renin secretion.
- Describe the functions of the macula densa.
- Define tubuloglomerular feedback and describe the mechanism for tubuloglomerular feedback and autoregulation of glomerular filtration rate.
- State the origin of atrial natriuretic peptides, the stimulus for their secretion, and their effect on sodium reabsorption and glomerular filtration rate.
- Describe the origin of antidiuretic hormone and the major controls of its secretion.

THE GOALS OF REGULATION

Total body sodium balance is crucially important to terrestrial animals. Because it is so important, overlapping and often redundant mechanisms have evolved to regulate total body sodium. As an example of this redundancy, neural input plays a significant role in regulating sodium transport, yet denervation of the kidneys or renal transplant does not abolish the ability of the kidneys to regulate sodium excretion. In addition, the specifics of how sodium is regulated depend on the simultaneous regulation of other substances. Although regulation of sodium excretion is admittedly complex, we can greatly simplify a description of this regulation by realizing there is a limited, and highly logical set of goals that these regulatory pathways accomplish. By focusing on these goals it is far easier to fit the details into the "big picture."

While everything the kidneys do is important in the long run, the immediate goal of regulating sodium and water is to promote the proper functioning of the cardiovascular system. But it must do so without compromising the regulation of other substances and the excretion of organic waste. The kidneys promote functioning of the cardiovascular system by maintaining ECF volume and keeping ECF osmolality within narrow limits. Since volume is almost entirely accounted for by water, and most of the ECF solute is sodium and its anions, the task of maintaining ECF volume and osmolality boils down to the co-regulation of sodium and water. Later in this chapter we will explore the cardiovascular connection in more detail; but for now we wish to present a general principle governing how the nephron as a whole regulates sodium excretion.

The kidneys always filter far more sodium than is excreted, and it might seem logical to control sodium excretion by varying the amount filtered, that is, vary GFR. While GFR is not absolutely constant, variation in GFR is not a major mechanism to regulate sodium excretion. The total amount of filtrate produced each day, and hence the amount of sodium entering the tubule, is kept within limits regardless of whether the body is conserving or getting rid of excess sodium. This constancy ensures that variations in sodium excretion do not interfere with the filtration of organic waste and substances other than sodium. The majority of sodium reabsorption occurs in the proximal tubule and thick ascending limb, that is, prior to the distal nephron. Not only is the amount filtered kept within limits, the amount reabsorbed early on is also regulated, so that the amount presented to the distal nephron does not vary greatly. As developed in the next section, much of the signaling to control GFR and proximal reabsorption comes from within the kidney itself and does not require external signaling. This then allows regulation of distal nephron sodium reabsorption to be responsive to cardiovascular needs and be the main target of *external* controls. So we can state the goals of regulating sodium transport to be (1) keep GFR within narrow limits, (2) keep the amount of sodium presented to the distal nephron also within narrow limits, and (3) vary distal nephron sodium reabsorption in response to signals that maintain total ECF volume and osmolality.

Regulation of GFR: Tubuloglomerular Feedback and the Macula Densa

The first regulatory task is to stabilize GFR. In Chapter 2 we discussed the autoregulation of GFR, which is partly a myogenic response to changes in renal artery pressure, and partly a feedback system that helps stabilize the amount of sodium presented to the distal nephron. The feedback system begins with the macula densa, which is a detector of tubular flow and sodium concentration. The macula densa is a component of the juxtaglomerular (jg) apparatus (see Figure 7–1). Besides helping regulate GFR, the macula densa is also a major player in the renin-angiotensin-aldosterone system described in detail later in this chapter. Regulation of GFR by the macula densa is called *tubuloglomerular feedback* (TG feedback), meaning from the tubule to the glomerulus. How does it work? The macula densa is located at the end of the loop of Henle where the tubule passes between the afferent and efferent arterioles of Bowman's capsule. It is able to sense (1) flow and (2) salt content in the tubular lumen. These are the net result of filtration and reabsorption in tubular elements preceding it, that is, the macula densa senses "everything done so far." Flow is sensed by cilia

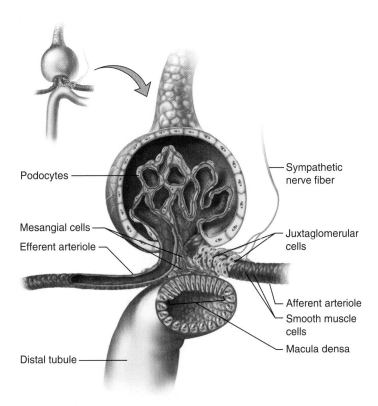

Podocytes

Sympathetic
nerve fiber

Mesangial cells

Efferent arteriole

Juxtaglomerular
cells

Afferent arteriole

Smooth muscle
cells

Macula densa

Distal tubule

Figure 7–1. The juxtaglomerular apparatus (jg apparatus). It is made up of (1) juxtaglomerular cells (granular cells), which are specialized smooth muscle cells surrounding the afferent arteriole, (2) extraglomerular mesangial cells, and (3) cells of the macula densa, which are part of the tubule. The close proximity of these components to each other permits chemical mediators released from one cell to easily diffuse to other components. Note that sympathetic nerve fibers innervate the granular cells. (Reproduced with permission from Widmaier EP, Raff H, Strang KT. *Vander's Human Physiology.* 11th ed. New York: McGraw-Hill; 2008.)

that project into the tubular lumen from macula densa cells. Bending of the cilia initiates intracellular signaling that leads to release of paracrine mediators. Tubular sodium chloride is sensed by uptake via N-K-2Cl multiporters whose action changes ionic concentrations within the macula densa cells and also causes release of paracrine mediators. When tubular flow and sodium content are high it is as if "the body has too much sodium" and "GFR is too high." The mediators released by the macula densa reduce GFR (restoring GFR to an appropriate level). The immediate mediator is ATP or its metabolite adenosine which bind to purinergic receptors on afferent arteriole smooth muscle. The subsequent rise in calcium in these cells stimulates contraction, thus reducing pressure and flow through the glomerular capillaries and reducing GFR.

What happens in the opposite case, that is, when there is low flow and low salt content flowing past the macula densa? Now "the body has too little sodium" and

"GFR is too low." This initiates the release of different mediators, specifically prostaglandins (e.g., PGE_2) and nitric oxide (NO). In the afferent arteriole NO is a dilator of smooth muscle. The effect is to raise flow and pressure in the glomerular capillaries and restore GFR to an appropriate level.

> *Tubuloglomerular feedback **dampens** changes in GFR caused by other controllers.*

The TG feedback mechanism acts on individual nephrons, that is, each macula densa feeds back only to the afferent arteriole supplying that nephron's glomerulus. This keeps filtration within an acceptable range while allowing other controllers to modify how much of the filtered sodium is ultimately reabsorbed. TG feedback doesn't initiate overall changes in GFR or prevent changes, rather it *dampens* changes originating from other signaling systems so that GFR doesn't vary "too much." Keep in mind that changes in GFR affect not only sodium, but every other filtered substance, and the kidneys have to maintain appropriate filtration in order to avoid deleterious effects on the excretion of those other substances.

Glomerulotubular Balance

Glomerulotubular balance (not to be confused with TG feedback described previously) refers to the phenomenon whereby sodium reabsorption in the proximal tubule varies in parallel with the filtered load, such that about two-thirds of the filtered sodium is reabsorbed even when GFR varies. Consider a 20% increase in GFR. If the reabsorbed amount remained fixed, all the excess would *not* be reabsorbed and would be passed on to the loop of Henle, an increase of 60%. But with glomerulotubular balance the amount reabsorbed also rises 20%, keeping the fractional reabsorption at two-thirds and limiting the rise in amount passed on to 20%. The mechanism by which reabsorption varies with filtered load appears to be via mechano-transduction by the microvilli on the apical surface of the proximal tubule cells, similar in principle to mechano-transduction by primary cilia in the macula densa. As flow changes, the amount of bending of the microvilli changes, and this is converted by cellular mechanisms into changes in transport. Be aware that two-thirds is only a rough approximation. The various controllers of sodium excretion operating in the proximal tubule are still functioning. In other words, sometimes exactly two-thirds of the filtered load is reabsorbed. At other times, it might be somewhat more or somewhat less, but the variation except under extremes of body conditions is limited. Figure 7–2 depicts the actions of TG feedback and GT balance to keep the amount of sodium leaving the proximal tubule relatively constant.

Sodium Excretion: The Cardiovascular Connection

We have emphasized that the kidneys work in partnership with the CV system. The kidneys maintain blood volume, regulate plasma osmolality, and secrete mediators that affect both cardiac performance and vascular tone (see Figure 7–3).

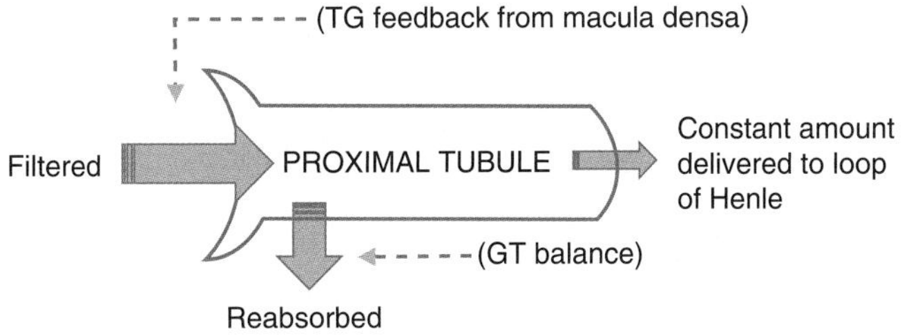

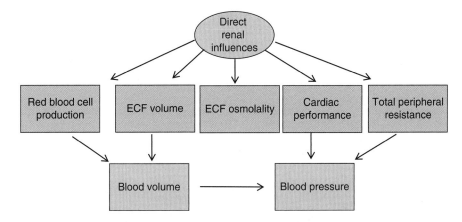

Figure 7–2. TG feedback and GT balance keep the amount of sodium filtered and reabsorbed in the proximal tubule within tight limits so that the amount delivered to the loop of Henle is nearly constant.

Figure 7–3. Influence of the kidneys on the cardiovascular system. The kidneys affect blood volume via their production of erythropoietin, which stimulates red blood cell production, and via their control of salt and water excretion. They also influence total peripheral resistance and cardiac performance via the actions of angiotensin II (see text for details). The combination of these factors affects blood pressure.

In turn, the CV system generates the pressure necessary for glomerular filtration and drives the high blood flow needed to maintain a stable cortical interstitial solute composition. Blood is composed primarily of red blood cells (about 45%) and blood plasma (about 55%). The kidneys are crucial for both parts—they secrete the hormone erythropoietin, which stimulates production of red blood cells, and they regulate the extracellular fluid (ECF) volume, of which blood plasma is a significant part

> *The kidneys partner with the CV system. The CV system provides the high pressure needed to drive glomerular filtration; the kidneys maintain the blood volume necessary to fill the vascular tree.*

(see Figure 6–1). On a short-term basis, circulating blood volume is kept constant in two ways. First, the splanchnic vascular beds vary their blood content to keep the amount circulating in the rest of the body more or less constant. Second, fluid moves between the vascular and interstitial spaces. Thus we can transiently take in excess fluids, or donate a unit of blood without a major effect on circulating blood volume. But in the long run, red blood cell mass and ECF volume cannot vary to extremes, and it is the job of the kidneys to keep both within acceptable limits.

Although ECF volume is set by its water content, sodium plays a crucial role in determining the amount of water it contains. In order to maintain osmolality, water in the ECF must track the amount of sodium. We can illustrate this concept numerically. ECF osmolality is approximated as follows:

$$\text{ECF osmolality} = \frac{\text{ECF solute content}}{\text{ECF volume}} \qquad \text{Equation 7-1}$$

By rearrangement this expression becomes:

$$\text{ECF volume} = \frac{\text{ECF solute content}}{\text{ECF osmolality}} \qquad \text{Equation 7-2}$$

Furthermore, since almost all of the ECF solute is accounted for by sodium and an equivalent number of anions (mostly chloride and bicarbonate), the amount of ECF solute is approximately twice the sodium content. We can write the previous expression as:

$$\text{ECF volume} \approx \frac{2 \times \text{Na content}}{\text{ECF osmolality}} \qquad \text{Equation 7-3}$$

To the extent that ECF osmolality is held within tight limits, ECF volume therefore varies directly with sodium content.

The preceding should not obscure the fact that osmolality does indeed vary. For example, drinking a large amount of pure water lowers osmolality, while sustained sweating on a hot day raises it. But deviations in osmolality are normally corrected much faster than are sodium loads. A pure water load is excreted within hours, while a deficit can be made up quickly by drinking fluids. Sodium loads, on the other hand, take days to excrete and sodium loads are associated with longer periods of volume excess.

Mechanisms to Assess ECF Sodium

Given the preceding information, the body requires methods to detect ECF volume and osmolality, and a system of effectors to regulate excretion of sodium and water in response to changes in one or both. Important afferent signals originate from pressures within the heart and vasculature, and osmolality in the CNS. There are also detectors of plasma sodium concentration in the CNS. This allows the body to differentiate between volume loads of pure water and volume loads containing sodium. We will describe osmoreception and the control of water excretion later in this chapter, and focus on sodium next.

Sodium concentration is detected by glial cells in regions of the brain called the circumventricular organs (described later in this chapter). They express sensory channels (Na_x) that respond to and act as detectors of extracellular sodium concentration. The glial cells modulate the activity of nearby neurons involved in the control of body sodium. There are also neurons in the hypothalamus containing sodium channels that respond to the sodium concentration in the cerebrospinal fluid. Thus, cells in or near the hypothalamus monitor extracellular sodium concentration.

Vascular Baroreceptors

Vascular pressures are assessed by *baroreceptors*—cells that deform in response to changes in local intravascular pressure. Three sets of baroreceptors are involved in controlling sodium excretion (see Figure 7–4). These are (1) arterial baroreceptors, nerve cells that mediate the classic baroreceptor reflex, (2) cardiopulmonary baroreceptors that are also nerve cells and work in parallel with the arterial baroreceptors, and (3) *intrarenal* baroreceptors, which are not nerve cells. We will describe the operation of intrarenal baroreceptors shortly. Of the three sets of baroreceptors, cardiopulmonary baroreceptors are the most important in normal circumstances. They have sensory endings located in the cardiac atria and parts of the pulmonary vasculature and serve as de facto blood volume detectors in the sense that pressures in the atria and pulmonary vessels rise

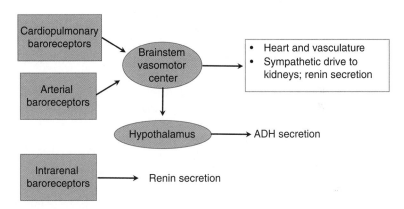

Figure 7–4. Baroreceptors and the major processes they influence. Cardiopulmonary baroreceptors sense pressure in the cardiac atria and pulmonary arteries, thereby being responsive to the filling of the vascular tree. They send afferent information to the brainstem vasomotor center, which then regulates cardiovascular and renal processes via autonomic efferents. Arterial baroreceptors sense pressures in the aorta and carotid arteries and send afferent information in parallel with the arterial baroreceptors. While there is overlap between the influences of the two sets of baroreceptors, the cardiopulmonary baroreceptors have a particularly important influence on the hypothalamus, which regulates secretion of ADH. The intrarenal baroreceptors have a major role in the renin-angiotensin system (see text for details).

when blood volume increases and fall when blood volume decreases. They send afferent neural information to the central nervous system. Arterial baroreceptors are located in the carotid arteries and arch of the aorta and sense pressure on a beat-by-beat basis. They also send afferent neural information to the central nervous system.

Information from neural baroreceptors is directed to a center for vascular control consisting of nuclei in the medulla oblongata (lower region of the brainstem close to where the brainstem merges with the spinal cord). Collectively these nuclei are called the *vasomotor center*. The vasomotor center stimulates vascular tone (vasoconstriction) throughout the body via the sympathetic nervous system, including the kidneys, as well as activating the renin-angiotensin system discussed below. In the arterioles of the peripheral vasculature this sympathetic tone maintains total peripheral resistance, and in the peripheral venous system it maintains central venous pressure via its ability to lower the compliance of large veins. By altering venous constriction in different vascular beds the vasomotor center can shift blood volume between the splanchnic organs and the circulating component. The vasomotor center also sends both sympathetic stimulatory and parasympathetic inhibitory signals to the heart. Baroreceptors exert tonic *inhibition* of the medullary vasomotor center, resulting in a brake on sympathetic drive. Increased pressures cause greater firing of the baroreceptors, more inhibition, and therefore less sympathetic drive to the periphery, while decreased pressures reduce firing in the baroreceptors and less inhibition, allowing more sympathetic drive. The neural signals to the heart, arterioles, and large veins change very rapidly when pressures fluctuate as a result of muscle activity or simple changes in posture. The result is to stabilize arterial pressure at its set-point, the mean arterial pressure, which for most people is slightly less than 100 mm Hg. The set-point is not rigidly fixed, however; it varies during the day, depending on activity and levels of excitement, and decreases about 20% during sleep.[1]

The baroreceptor/sympathetic drive system described above is very effective in maintaining arterial pressure at the set-point. A major complication and area of uncertainty lies in the long-term control of blood pressure. The question of "what sets the set-point" cannot be answered with confidence.[2] However, it is clear that malfunction in the renal handling of sodium or malfunction in renal signaling can lead to hypertension. Any consideration of the long-term control of blood pressure must include renal actions.

Given the preceding discussion, we should emphasize two major points. First, while arterial blood pressure does influence renal sodium excretion, particularly in extreme circumstances such as circulatory shock, on a day-to-day basis it is ECF volume that has the more significant impact. Second, the description of neural

---

[1]As an example of this variation, some patients experience "white coat hypertension," an elevation of blood pressure that is manifested in response to the stress of being in a doctor's office.

[2]Arterial pressure is one among many physiological variables regulated around a set point, for example, body temperature, partial pressure of carbon dioxide, or plasma concentration of glucose. While much is known about the mechanisms that keep these variables close to their set-points, the question of "what sets their set-points" remains unclear.

mechanisms should not leave the mistaken impression that the nervous system has exclusive control over the kidneys. As mentioned earlier, transplanted kidneys with no neural connections can still regulate sodium excretion. Clearly there are other controls acting in parallel with neural signaling that allow the kidneys to regulate sodium excretion in ordinary circumstances.

MAJOR CONTROLLERS OF SODIUM EXCRETION

The Renin-Angiotensin System

The renin-angiotensin system is the major regulator of renal sodium excretion. It is a signaling pathway regulating multiple processes in the kidney and elsewhere, and is controlled in part by sympathetic neural signals influenced by vascular baroreceptors. What is traditionally described as *the* renin-angiotensin system is really a *set* of renin-angiotensin systems. There is both a system that leads to systemic circulating renin and angiotensin system, and separate intra-organ renin-angiotensin systems in many tissues, including, but not limited to, the heart, sex organs, brain, and the kidneys.

The system leading to circulating renin-angiotensin is intimately involved with controlling the steroid hormone aldosterone and is appropriately called the renin-angiotensin-aldosterone system (RAAS). It consists of a protein substrate (angiotensinogen), the enzyme renin that splits off a 10 amino acid peptide (angiotensin I) from angiotensinogen, several additional enzymes that split angiotensin I into smaller peptides, and finally receptors for the peptides that activate cellular actions upon binding. The most important of these smaller peptides is the eight amino acid peptide angiotensin II (AII). It is formed from angiotensin I by the action of angiotensin-converting enzyme (ACE). AII is a mediator of multiple effects in the kidneys and elsewhere and stimulates production of aldosterone.

In the circulating RAAS, angiotensinogen is synthesized in the liver (see Figure 7–5). Plasma angiotensinogen levels are normally high and not rate limiting. Furthermore, ACE, which is expressed on the endothelial surfaces of the vascular system, particularly the pulmonary vessels, avidly converts most of the angiotensin I into AII. Therefore, the major determinant of circulating AII is the amount of renin available to form angiotensin I. As outlined in Chapter 1 and shown in Figure 7–1, renin is produced by the jg apparatus. The renin-secreting cells are located in the late afferent arteriole just before the glomerulus, and are referred to as either jg cells or granular cells (because renin can be visualized as secretory granules).

The level of circulating renin varies inversely with dietary sodium. A high sodium diet suppresses renin secretion, while a low sodium diet leads to high levels of renin. The secretion of renin by the jg cells is under the control of three known regulators. The first is sympathetic input via the renal sympathetic nerve. Norepinephrine released from postganglionic sympathetic neurons acts on β_1-adrenergic receptors in the jg cells. This activates a c-AMP-mediated pathway that causes the release of renin. The jg cells are quite sensitive to norepinephrine and respond to low levels of sympathetic activity that may have minimal direct effect

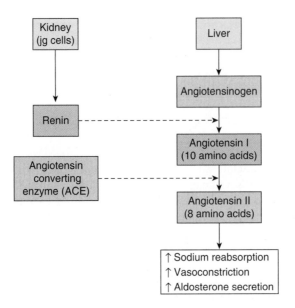

Figure 7–5. Major components and actions of the systemic RAAS. Renin is secreted by renal jg cells into the blood and acts on circulating angiotensinogen from the liver to produce angiotensin I. Most of the angiotensin I is converted to angiotensin II (AII) by angiotensin-converting enzyme (ACE) in the walls of the peripheral vasculature. AII has multiple actions, chief ones being a vasoconstrictor and stimulator of adrenal production of aldosterone. AII acts within the kidneys to promote sodium reabsorption.

on the renal vasculature or sodium transport. Sympathetic drive is highly influenced by feedback from the vasculature. Low vascular volume detected by cardiopulmonary baroreceptors pressures leads to increased sympathetic drive to the jg cells and increased release of renin, while high pressures suppress renin secretion.

The second controller of renin secretion is pressure in the afferent arteriole. The jg cells not only respond to vascular pressures indirectly via adrenergic stimulation, they respond *directly* to changes in afferent arteriolar pressure. When pressure in the afferent arteriole decreases, renin production increases. Except in cases of major renal arterial blockage, pressure in the arteriolar lumen at the jg cells is close to systemic arterial pressure and changes in parallel with it. Because the jg cells respond to vascular pressure they are acting as baroreceptors. In fact, the jg cells are the *intrarenal* baroreceptors mentioned previously. Even though they are not neurons and do not send afferent feedback, they are baroreceptors nevertheless. Consider what happens when there is a major drop in arterial pressure. The intrarenal baroreceptors (the jg cells) sense the drop in pressure and increase their secretion of renin. Simultaneously the fall in pressure is also sensed by the arterial baroreceptors in the carotid arteries and aorta. The decrease in their afferent signaling allows the vasomotor center to increase sympathetic drive to the jg cells, resulting in a huge combined stimulation of renin secretion.

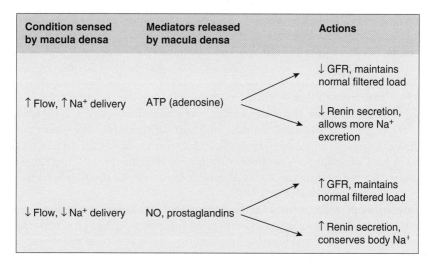

Condition sensed by macula densa	Mediators released by macula densa	Actions
↑ Flow, ↑ Na⁺ delivery	ATP (adenosine)	↓ GFR, maintains normal filtered load ↓ Renin secretion, allows more Na⁺ excretion
↓ Flow, ↓ Na⁺ delivery	NO, prostaglandins	↑ GFR, maintains normal filtered load ↑ Renin secretion, conserves body Na⁺

Figure 7–6. Feedback control by the macula densa. The macula densa, located at the end of the loop of Henle, senses both flow and sodium delivery. In response it modulates two different processes in parallel. First, tubuloglomerular feedback, which is a component of GFR autoregulation, blunts changes in GFR caused by other signals, thus keeping GFR within a narrow range. Second, the modulation of renin secretion helps maintain total body sodium, and thus the filtered load, at an acceptable level.

The third controller of renin release originates from another component of the jg apparatus; namely the macula densa, the function of which we previously described in terms of tubuloglomerular feedback. The macula densa is also a major player in the control of renin production and uses the same mediators that regulate contraction of the afferent arteriole. In response to high tubular sodium at the macula densa, adenosine (produced extracellularly from released ATP) binds to purinergic receptors on the nearby jg cells. This has the effect of increasing intracellular calcium and reducing the release of renin.[3] In turn, the reduction in renin secretion reduces the levels of AII and allows the kidneys to excrete more of the filtered sodium. In contrast, low tubular sodium at the macula densa releases NO and prostaglandins. In the jg cells the prostaglandins stimulate or prolong the lifetime of c-AMP, thereby stimulating the release of renin. The now-activated RAAS reduces sodium excretion. The operation of the macula densa in feedback control of the RAAS and GFR autoregulation is shown in Figure 7–6.

Finally, descriptions of the RAAS quite naturally focus on its activation and subsequent stimulation of sodium reabsorption. This is because retention of sodium is crucial during hypovolemic emergencies and in unusual circumstances when dietary sodium is not plentiful. However, on typical Western diets the salt

---

[3]In most secretory processes, for example, in nerve terminals, secretion of materials stored in secretory granules is stimulated by a rise in intracellular calcium. However, in jg cells, calcium inhibits secretion.

content of meals is often in excess, and it is imperative to let the kidneys excrete salt loads promptly. The main way this is accomplished is by decreasing the activity of the RAAS. Figure 7–7 summarizes control of renin secretion.

KEY ACTIONS OF AII

 Vasoconstriction—AII is a potent vasoconstrictor, acting on the vasculature of many peripheral tissues, the effect of which is to raise arterial pressure. It also vasoconstricts both cortical and medullary vessels in the kidney. This reduces total renal blood flow and reduces GFR, thus decreasing the filtered load of sodium. A number of drugs for the treatment of hypertension either reduce the production of AII (ACE inhibitors) or block the peripheral receptors for AII (see later discussion).

Stimulation of sodium tubular reabsorption—AII stimulates sodium reabsorption in both the proximal tubule and distal nephron. In the proximal tubule it stimulates the NHE3 sodium/hydrogen antiporter in the apical membrane and the Na-K-ATPase in the basolateral membrane. In the distal tubule and connecting tubule it stimulates the activity of NCC sodium/chloride symporters and sodium channels (ENaC) that import sodium. Its actions in the proximal tubule are normally overridden by the intrarenal feedback controls described earlier in this chapter.

Stimulation of the CNS: salt appetite, thirst, and sympathetic drive—AII stimulates behavioral actions in response to fluid loss that increase salt appetite and thirst. AII acts on the circumventricular organs in the brain that are described later in this chapter. These function as detectors of many substances in the blood and convey information to various areas of the brain. In situations of volume depletion and low blood pressure, when circulating levels of AII are high, a key effect, in addition to vascular and tubular actions, is increased thirst and salt appetite. These pathways also increase sympathetic drive.

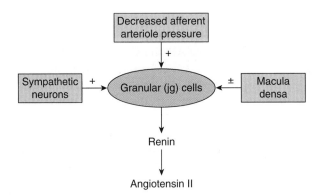

Figure 7–7. Control of renin secretion. Sympathetic stimulation and decreased afferent arteriole pressure both stimulate renin secretion. Paracrine agents released by the macula densa either stimulate or inhibit renin release depending on circumstances as discussed in the text.

> *Angiotensin II is a very important agent to preserve blood volume and blood pressure. It directly stimulates sodium reabsorption, stimulates aldosterone secretion, and causes general vasoconstriction.*

⑦ Stimulation of aldosterone secretion—Aldosterone is a major stimulator of sodium reabsorption in the distal nephron, that is, regions of the tubule *beyond* the proximal tubule and loop of Henle. Aldosterone-stimulated sodium retention is an effector system that is vital in correcting prolonged reductions in body sodium, blood pressure, and volume. We focus here on the role of aldosterone in sodium reabsorption, but aldosterone has many other important actions, including stimulation of potassium excretion and acid excretion (see Chapters 8 and 9).

The most important physiological factor controlling secretion of aldosterone is the circulating level of AII, which stimulates the adrenal cortex to secrete aldosterone. This targets the distal nephron to increase sodium reabsorption and thus increase total body sodium and blood volume to produce a long-term correction to total body sodium content.

The main cellular targets of aldosterone are cells in the distal tubule and beyond. An action on these cells is what one would expect for fine-tuning the output of sodium, because most of the filtered sodium has already been reabsorbed in prior segments.

As a molecule, aldosterone has enough lipid character to freely cross tubular cell membranes, after which it combines with mineralocorticoid receptors in the cytoplasm. Aldosterone binding promotes transport of the receptor to the nucleus where it acts as a transcription factor that promotes gene expression of specific proteins. In principal cells of the connecting tubule the effect of these proteins is to increase the activity of sodium channels (ENaCs) and basolateral membrane Na-K-ATPase pumps. And when the level of AII is elevated aldosterone also promotes the activity of luminal NCC sodium/chloride symporters in the distal tubule. Thus, the major pathways for sodium reabsorption are stimulated (Figure 7–8). However, without the simultaneous presence of AII, aldosterone is not very effective at stimulating NCC activity and promoting sodium reabsorption. Under these conditions aldosterone still plays a major role in regulating potassium secretion (see Chapter 8).

The percentage of sodium reabsorption dependent on the influence of aldosterone is approximately 2% of the filtered load. Thus, all other factors remaining constant, in the complete absence of aldosterone, a person would excrete 2% of the filtered sodium, whereas in the presence of high plasma concentrations of aldosterone, virtually no sodium would be excreted. Two percent of the filtered sodium may seem trivial but is actually a significant amount because so much sodium is filtered:

$$\text{Total filtered sodium/day} = \text{GFR} \times \text{plasma Na} \qquad \text{Equation 7-4}$$
$$= 180 \text{ L/day} \times 140 \text{ mmol/L}$$
$$= 25{,}200 \text{ mmol/day}$$

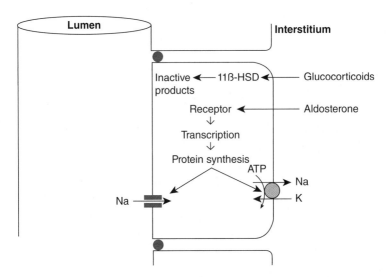

Figure 7–8. Mechanism of aldosterone action. Aldosterone enters principal cells and interacts with cytosolic aldosterone receptors. The aldosterone-bound receptors interact with nuclear DNA to promote gene expression. The aldosterone-induced gene products activate sodium channels in the apical membrane and sodium pumps in the basolateral membrane, causing increased sodium reabsorption. Glucocorticoids such as cortisol are also capable of binding to the aldosterone receptor. However, they are inactivated by 11β-hydroxysteroid dehydrogenase (11β-HSD).

Thus, aldosterone controls the reabsorption of $0.02 \times 25,200$ mmol/day $= 504$ mmol/day. In terms of sodium chloride, the form in which most sodium is ingested, this amounts to the control of almost 30 g NaCl/day, an amount considerably more than the average person consumes. Therefore, by control of the plasma concentration of aldosterone between minimal and maximal, the excretion of sodium can be finely adjusted to the intake so that total body sodium remains constant.

Aldosterone also stimulates sodium transport by other epithelia in the body, namely, sweat and salivary ducts and the intestine. The net effect is the same as that exerted on the kidney: movement of sodium from lumen to blood. Thus, aldosterone is an all-purpose stimulator of sodium retention.

AII produced by the circulating RAAS system is a major stimulator of aldosterone secretion. Since levels of angiotensin II are controlled by renin, this emphasizes the importance of renin in the control of sodium reabsorption. Both renin and aldosterone have relatively short plasma half-lives (~15 minutes), while the half-life of angiotensin II is very short (<1 minute). Therefore, prolonged action of aldosterone requires the continuous stimulation of renin secretion and production of AII.

An elevated plasma potassium concentration is also a stimulator of aldosterone secretion, and depletion of potassium is an inhibitor, and may in some cases counteract the stimulating effect of AII. We will address this topic in Chapter 8. Atrial natriuretic factors (discussed later) also inhibit aldosterone secretion.

Table 7–1. Actions of angiotensin II that cause sodium retention and directly or indirectly increase blood pressure

Stimulates sodium reabsorption in proximal tubule (NHE and Na-K-ATPase)
Stimulates sodium reabsorption in distal tubule (Na-Cl symporter)
Stimulates sodium reabsorption in collecting tubule (ENac channels)
Stimulates constriction of afferent arteriole (decreases GFR)
Stimulates secretion of aldosterone
Stimulates sympathetic outflow from CNS
Stimulates general peripheral vasoconstriction

From all of the preceding discussion it should be clear that AII is a hugely important agent to preserve blood volume and blood pressure. It does so by retaining sodium, both through its own actions and via aldosterone, and by causing general vasoconstriction. The major actions of AII that lead to sodium retention and increased blood pressure are shown in Table 7–1. We will describe its influence on potassium excretion in Chapter 8.

MAJOR CONTROLLERS OF SODIUM EXCRETION

Sympathetic Stimulation

The sympathetic nervous system is capable of an emergency "fight-or-flight" response, but its normal operation is a differential modulation of various functions within different organs. The vasculature and tubules of the kidney are innervated by postganglionic sympathetic neurons that release norepinephrine. In most regions of the kidney norepinephrine is recognized by α-adrenergic receptors. In the renal vasculature activation of α_1-adrenergic receptors causes vasoconstriction of afferent and efferent arterioles. This reduces renal blood flow and GFR.

Quite obviously GFR is a crucial determinant of sodium excretion. Without filtration, there is no excretion. However, except in body emergencies such as hypovolemic shock, GFR is kept within rather narrow limits due to autoregulation. Thus, while neural control does affect GFR, this component of sympathetic control is probably not important in normal circumstances. Neural control of the renal vasculature is exerted primarily on blood flow in the cortex, allowing preservation of medullary perfusion even when cortical blood flow is reduced.

The proximal tubule epithelial cells are innervated by α_1- and α_2-adrenergic receptors. Stimulation of these receptors in the proximal tubule by norepinephrine activates both components of the main transcellular sodium reabsorptive pathway, that is, the sodium-hydrogen antiporter NHE3 in the apical membrane and the Na-K-ATPase in the basolateral membrane. This pathway is activated in emergency situations in which it is appropriate to reduce sodium excretion, for example, volume depletion or low blood pressure.

> *Sympathetic stimulation stimulates sodium reabsorption in the proximal tubule and reduces renal blood flow and GFR.*

The effects of sympathetic stimulation on cells in the distal nephron are less straightforward. Other agonists are co-released with norepinephrine and affect other receptor types (e.g., ATP acting on purinergic receptors). However, the overall influence of sympathetic stimulation of the kidney is reduced sodium excretion.

Modulation of Sodium Excretion: Dopamine

Activation of the regulators described in the preceding sections, that is, sympathetic input, AII, and aldosterone, all serve to increase sodium reabsorption. Another major regulator is dopamine, but its action is different—namely it *inhibits* sodium reabsorption. Dopamine is generally known as a neurotransmitter in the central nervous system that participates in multiple functions including the control of body movement. The dopamine that acts in the kidney is not released from neurons, rather it is synthesized in proximal tubule cells from the precursor L-DOPA (the same substance employed in the treatment of Parkinsonism). L-DOPA is taken up from the renal circulation and glomerular filtrate and converted to dopamine in the proximal tubule epithelium, and then released to act in a paracrine manner on nearby cells. Although the signaling path is not clear, it is known that increases in sodium intake lead to increased production of intrarenal dopamine. Dopamine has two actions, both of which reduce sodium reabsorption. First, it causes internalization of NHE antiporters and Na-K-ATPase pumps into intracellular vesicles, thereby reducing transcellular sodium reabsorption. Second, it reduces the expression of AII receptors, thereby decreasing the ability of AII to stimulate sodium reabsorption. Therefore, dopamine, in combination with sympathetic input and the RAAS, comprises a true push-pull system that exerts bidirectional control over sodium reabsorption.

Other Regulators and Influences on Sodium Excretion

Sympathetic input, the RAAS and dopamine are all means of regulating sodium excretion. As should be clear from the previous discussion, these processes influence each other, together yielding a final rate of sodium excretion that meets the goals outlined in the beginning of this chapter. There are still other signals and processes that contribute to regulation, some of which are outlined below.

ADH

We previously described the role of ADH in regulating the reabsorption of water in the collecting duct system and will address this topic again later in the chapter. ADH also plays a direct role in regulating sodium excretion. When ADH binds to V2 receptors in tubular cells it increases the production of c-AMP. This results in increased activity of the NKCC multiporter in the thick ascending limb and increased numbers of sodium channels (ENaC) in principal cells of the distal nephron, thereby increasing the uptake of sodium which, in both regions, is actively transported into the interstitium by the Na-K-ATPase. Interestingly, in the distal nephron the mechanism proceeds, not by moving ENaCs into the membrane, but rather by decreasing their removal and degradation. As mentioned in Chapter 4, transport proteins have a finite lifetime in membranes before being degraded. A process that slows degradation of a transport protein has the same effect as increasing the expression and insertion of the protein.

PRESSURE NATRIURESIS AND DIURESIS

Because the kidneys are responsive to arterial pressure there are situations in which elevated blood pressure can lead directly to increased excretion of sodium, particularly if the body contains excess fluid. This phenomenon is called pressure natriuresis, and because natriuresis is usually accompanied by water (see later discussion), it is often called pressure diuresis. This is an intrarenal phenomenon, not requiring external signaling. However, external signals normally override pressure natriuresis, as occurs, for example, in aerobic exercise when arterial pressure is somewhat increased, but sodium excretion is decreased. In addition, a common cause of hypertension is renal pathology that inappropriately activates the intrarenal RAS. In these cases, the elevated arterial pressure fails to increase sodium excretion.

NATRIURETIC PEPTIDES

Several tissues in the body synthesize members of a hormone family called *natriuretic peptides*, so named because they promote excretion of sodium in the urine. Key among these are atrial (ANP) and brain natriuretic peptide (BNP; named as such because it was first discovered in the brain). The main source of both natriuretic peptides is the heart. The natriuretic peptides have both vascular and tubular actions. They relax the afferent arteriole, thereby promoting increased filtration, and act at several sites in the tubule. They inhibit release of renin, inhibit the actions of angiotensin II that normally promote reabsorption of sodium, and act in the medullary collecting duct to inhibit sodium absorption. The major stimulus for increased secretion of the natriuretic peptides is distention of the atria, which occurs during plasma volume expansion. This is probably the stimulus for the increased natriuretic peptides that occurs in persons on a high-salt diet. Although most experts assume that these peptides play some physiological role in the regulation of sodium excretion in this and other situations in which plasma volume is expanded, it is not currently possible to quantitate precisely their contribution, although it is surely less than aldosterone. These peptides are greatly elevated in patients with heart failure and can serve as diagnostic indicators.

Summary of the Control of Sodium Excretion

Sodium excretion is controlled by interacting signaling systems that include intrarenal mechanisms and external signals relating to the CV system (Figure 7–9). The main overall goal is to preserve a total mass of sodium in the ECF that maintains appropriate osmotic content for the CV system, but without compromising the excretion of other substances. Intrarenal mechanisms keep the amount of sodium

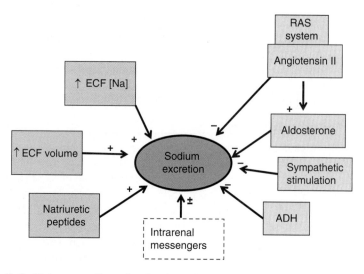

Figure 7–9. Major controllers of sodium excretion. Controllers on the left side increase sodium excretion, while controllers on the right side inhibit sodium excretion. A major means to increase sodium excretion is to decrease activity of the controllers that stimulate sodium reabsorption, particularly the RAAS system. Intrarenal controls both stimulate and inhibit sodium excretion.

filtered and the amount reabsorbed in the proximal tubule within narrow limits, leaving control of the amount excreted to signals acting on the distal nephron, particularly sodium channels in the collecting duct system and sodium-chloride cotransporters in the distal tubule. The most important signaling system is the RAAS which has both intrarenal and extrarenal aspects. Plasma renin levels vary inversely with dietary sodium, thereby either stimulating recovery of the sodium entering the distal nephron or allowing it to be excreted. Important detection systems include baroreceptors in various locations, cells in the CNS that detect sodium concentration, and intrarenal sensors of tubular sodium concentration and flow. Neural baroreceptors respond to pressures in the heart and pulmonary circuit, thereby providing information about volume, while arterial baroreceptor and intrarenal baroreceptors give information about arterial pressure. Under all circumstances, even with considerable excess dietary sodium, the vast majority of filtered sodium (over 98%) is reabsorbed, but because so much sodium is filtered, even small adjustments in reabsorption result in large cumulative changes in total body sodium.

CONTROL OF WATER EXCRETION

 Water excretion, as with sodium excretion, is regulated in partnership with the CV system. Central goals in regulating both salt and water excretion are to (1) preserve vascular volume and (2) maintain plasma osmolality at a level that is healthy for tissue cells. The main regulators of water excretion, not surprisingly, relate to osmolality and volume.

Quantitatively, renal water excretion is determined by two values: (1) the amount of solute in the urine and (2) the osmolality of the urine.

$$\text{Urine water excretion} = \frac{\text{urine solute excretion}}{\text{urine osmolality}} \qquad \text{Equation 7-5}$$

Excreted solute consists mostly of organic waste and excess electrolytes. In a given metabolic state, the rate of organic waste excretion is more or less constant, and is not altered for purposes of controlling water excretion. Electrolyte excretion is highly regulated, but more to achieve balance of individual substances like sodium and potassium than to control water excretion per se. Given that solute excretion is so variable, the main way the body controls water excretion in normal circumstances is to control urine osmolality. In other words, given a certain amount of solute that is excreted, the body controls the amount of water accompanying it by controlling urine osmolality.

When the body excretes urine that is more dilute than plasma (osmolality below 285 mOsm/kg H_2O), the body is excreting "free water" (like adding pure water to otherwise isosmotic urine). Conversely, when the excreted urine is more concentrated than plasma, there is "negative free water" excretion. It is as if the body has reclaimed pure water from otherwise isosmotic urine.

As we already know from Chapter 6 the kidneys first generate hypo-osmotic tubular fluid in the loop of Henle. Then as the fluid subsequently flows through the collecting duct system, variable amounts of water are reabsorbed by allowing the tubular fluid to equilibrate to varying degrees with the surrounding interstitium. The final osmolality, and hence final volume, depends on the peak medullary osmolality and how closely the tubular osmolality approaches that value. We also know that equilibration with the interstitium is a function of water permeability in the collecting ducts under the control of the hormone ADH. Therefore, the regulation of water excretion that is *independent* of solute excretion focuses on controls over ADH secretion.

Water excretion varies in proportion to solute excretion and inversely with urine osmolality.

ADH (also called arginine vasopressin because of its role as a vasoconstrictor) is a small peptide (nine amino acids) synthesized by neurons in the hypothalamus. The cell bodies are located in the supraoptic and paraventricular nuclei of the hypothalamus. Their axons extend downward to the posterior pituitary gland, from which ADH is released into the blood. There is normally a moderate rate of ADH secretion, allowing considerable water reabsorption in the renal collecting ducts, and resulting in urine that is more concentrated than plasma. ADH secretion can increase or decrease from this level, giving the control system a bidirectional responsiveness. And because the collecting ducts are very sensitive to ADH, this allows the body to control water excretion rate over a very wide range. There are many sources of synaptic input to the ADH-secreting neurons. The most important signals originate in osmorecep-tors and CV baroreceptors.

Osmoreceptor Control of ADH Secretion

Plasma osmolality is one of the most tightly regulated variables in the body. Plasma osmolality is set mainly by the ratio of ECF sodium (plus its associated anions) to water. Other solutes (e.g., glucose and potassium) make some contribution, but those other solutes are regulated for reasons other than their effect on plasma osmolality. Thus, except under unusual circumstances such as severe hyperglycemia, variations in plasma osmolality mostly reflect varia-tions in sodium concentration. If the body keeps the inputs and outputs of sodium and water matched in lock step, osmolality remains constant. But inputs are often *not* matched. The major effect of gaining or losing water or salt without corre-sponding changes in the other is a change in the osmolality of the body fluids. When osmolality deviates from normal, strong reflexes come into play to change ADH secretion, and thus change the excretion of water.

Key receptors that initiate reflexes controlling ADH secretion are *osmoreceptors*, neurons responsive to changes in osmolality. Most osmoreceptors are located in tissues surrounding the third cerebral ventricle. These tissues, along with those surrounding the fourth cerebral ventricle, are known collectively as *circumven-tricular organs*. While the vast majority of cerebral tissue is separated from direct contact with substances in the blood by impermeability of the vascular endothe-lium (the blood-brain barrier), the circumventricular organs contain fenestrated capillaries. The fenestrations allow rapid adjustment of local interstitial composi-tion when plasma composition changes. Osmoreceptors shrink and swell in response to changes in local osmolality. This affects the activity of stretch-sensitive channels in their membranes, which thereby transduce osmotic changes into elec-trical signals. The hypothalamic cells that synthesize ADH receive synaptic input from osmoreceptors in the circumventricular organs. Via these connections, an increase in osmolality increases the rate of ADH secretion. In turn, this causes water permeability of the collecting ducts to increase, water reabsorption rises, and a small volume of concentrated (hyperosmotic) urine is excreted. By excreting solute in excess of water, body fluid osmolality decreases toward normal. Conversely, decreased plasma osmolality inhibits ADH secretion. For example, when a person drinks pure water, the excess water lowers the body fluid osmolal-ity, which inhibits ADH secretion. As a result, water permeability of the collecting ducts becomes low, little water is reabsorbed from these segments, and a large volume of dilute (hypo-osmotic) urine is excreted. In this manner, the excess water is rapidly eliminated and plasma osmolality is increased (see Figure 7–10).

Osmoreceptors in tissues surrounding cerebral ventricles stimulate ADH secretion when osmolality rises.

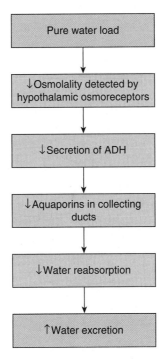

Figure 7–10. Mechanism for increased water excretion in response to a pure water load. Decreased plasma osmolality leads, via osmoreceptors, to decreased secretion of ADH (vasopressin), in turn causing decreased collecting duct water reabsorption and more water excretion.

Earlier we mentioned specific sodium-detecting glial cells located in the circumventricular organs and hypothalamic neurons that contain Na_x channels. The amount of ADH that is secreted at a given level of plasma osmolality is modulated by information about sodium concentration detected in these cells. Most of the time the influence on ADH secretion from sodium-detecting cells and osmoreceptors is synergistic (i.e., both high sodium concentration and high osmolality stimulate ADH).

The osmoreceptor-ADH system is very sensitive, responding to an osmolality change of only 1 or 2 mOsm/kg. However, common perturbations are often a good deal greater than this. For example, if a 70-kg person consumes 1 L of pure water, ECF osmolality is reduced by about 7 mOsm/kg. And exercise for several hours on a warm day can increase ECF osmolality by 10 mOsm/kg or more. Such routine perturbations result in strong ADH responses that remain active until osmolality returns to its previous value. ADH has a plasma half-life of only a few minutes, so prolonged stimulation of water permeability in the kidneys requires continuous stimulation of the ADH-secreting neurons.

Baroreceptor Control of ADH Secretion

There is another major influence on ADH secretion. This originates in systemic baroreceptors (the same ones that influence sympathetic drive to the kidneys). A decreased extracellular volume or major decrease in arterial pressure reflexively activates increased ADH secretion. The response is mediated by neural pathways originating in cardiopulmonary baroreceptors, and if arterial pressure decreases, from arterial baroreceptors.

Decreased CV pressures cause less firing by the baroreceptors, which relieves inhibition of stimulatory pathways and results in more ADH secretion. In effect, the low CV pressures are interpreted as low volume, and the response of increased ADH appropriately serves to minimize loss of water (see Figure 7–11). Conversely, baroreceptors are stimulated by increased CV pressures, interpreted as excess volume, and this causes inhibition of ADH secretion. The decrease in ADH results in decreased reabsorption of water in the collecting ducts, and more excretion. The adaptive value of these baroreceptor reflexes is to help stabilize ECF volume and ultimately blood pressure.

There is a second adaptive value to this reflex: Large decreases in plasma volume, as might occur after a major hemorrhage, elicit such high concentrations of

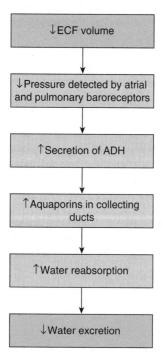

Figure 7–11. Decreased water excretion in response to decreased plasma volume. Low pressure is sensed by neural baroreceptors. Their reduced firing removes inhibition of the hypothalamic cells whose axons release ADH (vasopressin) from the posterior pituitary gland. The subsequent increase in ADH increases water reabsorption in the collecting ducts and helps preserve existing volume.

ADH—much higher than those needed to produce maximal antidiuresis—that the hormone is able to exert direct vasoconstrictor effects on arteriolar smooth muscle. The result is increased total peripheral resistance, which helps restore arterial blood pressure independently of the slower restoration of body fluid volume. Renal arterioles also participate in this constrictor response, and so a high plasma concentration of ADH, quite apart from its effect on water permeability and sodium reabsorption in the distal nephron, promotes retention of both sodium and water by lowering GFR. In effect the body suspends the normal filtration of organic waste in order to deal with the immediate crisis of low blood volume.

We have described two different major afferent pathways controlling the ADH-secreting hypothalamic cells: one from baroreceptors and one from osmoreceptors. These hypothalamic cells are, therefore, true integrators, whose activity is determined by the total synaptic input to them. Thus, a simultaneous increase in plasma volume and decrease in body fluid osmolality causes strong inhibition of ADH secretion. Conversely, a simultaneous decrease in plasma volume and increase in osmolality produces very marked stimulation of ADH secretion. However, what happens when baroreceptor and osmoreceptor inputs oppose each other (e.g., if plasma volume and osmolality are both decreased)? In general, because of the high sensitivity of the osmoreceptors, the osmoreceptor influence predominates over that of the baroreceptors when changes in osmolality and plasma volume are small to moderate. However, a dangerous reduction in plasma volume will take precedence over decreased body fluid osmolality in influencing ADH secretion; under such conditions, water is retained in excess of solute even though the body fluids become hypo-osmotic (for the same reason, plasma sodium concentration decreases). In essence, when blood volume reaches a life-threatening low level, it is more important for the body to preserve vascular volume and thus ensure an adequate cardiac output than it is to preserve normal osmolality.

The cells that synthesize ADH in the hypothalamus also receive synaptic input from many other brain areas. Thus, ADH secretion and, hence, urine flow can be altered by pain, fear, and a variety of other factors, including drugs such as alcohol, which inhibits ADH release. However, the influence of these other factors should not obscure the generalization that ADH secretion is determined over the long term primarily by the states of body fluid osmolality and plasma volume.

Figure 7–12 shows the major factors known to control renal sodium and water excretion in response to severe sweating. Sweat is mainly a hypo-osmotic salt solution. Therefore, sweating causes both a decrease in ECF volume and an increase in body fluid osmolality. This strongly activates the RAAS and secretion of ADH, leading to increased reabsorption of both sodium and water. These responses interact with each other. First, the high levels of ADH aid in the reabsorption of sodium. Second, reducing sodium excretion reduces the osmotic load in the urine that obligates water to accompany it.

THIRST AND SALT APPETITE

Deficits of salt and water cannot be corrected by renal conservation, and ingestion is the ultimate compensatory mechanism. The subjective feeling of thirst, which drives

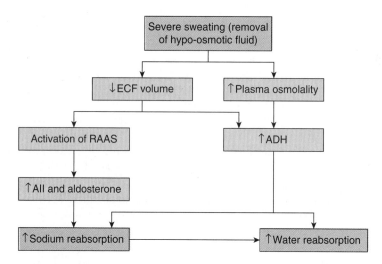

Figure 7–12. Coordinated response to severe sweating. The secretions of sweat glands produce a hypo-osmotic fluid, leaving the remaining body fluids decreased in volume and somewhat hyperosmotic. A combination of decreased ECF volume and increased plasma osmolality activates reflexes that preserve both salt and water.

one to obtain and ingest water, is stimulated both by reduced plasma volume and by increased body fluid osmolality. The adaptive significance of both is self-evident. Note that these are precisely the same changes that stimulate ADH production, and the receptors—osmoreceptors and the nerve cells that respond to the CV baroreceptors—that initiate the ADH-controlling reflexes are near those that initiate thirst. The thirst response, however, is significantly less sensitive than the ADH response.

There are also other pathways controlling thirst. For example, dryness of the mouth and throat causes profound thirst, which is relieved by merely moistening them. Also, when animals such as the camel (and humans, to a lesser extent) become markedly dehydrated, they will rapidly drink just enough water to replace their previous losses and then stop. What is amazing is that when they stop, the water has not yet had time to be absorbed from the gastrointestinal tract into the blood. Some kind of metering of the water intake by the gastrointestinal tract has occurred, but its nature remains a mystery. Neural afferents from the pharynx and upper gastrointestinal tract are likely to be involved.

Congestive Heart Failure and Hypertension: Cardiovascular Pathologies That Involve the Kidneys

 We conclude this chapter with a brief description of congestive heart failure and hypertension, two very common pathologies, particularly in the geriatric population. They both directly or indirectly involve the kidneys

---

[4]In contrast to atrial pressures that are high, *arterial* pressure is usually within the normal range, and heart failure cannot be diagnosed based on arterial blood pressure.

and illustrate the connections between the renal and CV systems, not only in normal function, but pathology as well. This is brought home by the fact that primary therapies for both pathologies employ drugs that alter renal function. In congestive heart failure and in most cases of hypertension, the perturbed function lies in inappropriate *signaling* to or within the kidneys rather than pathology of renal transport mechanisms per se.

Congestive heart failure occurs when cardiac muscle is weakened (for any of several reasons) and the heart becomes less effective as a pump. It cannot increase cardiac output to meet the demands of exercise and, more importantly, can only provide adequate resting cardiac output in the presence of excessive neurohumoral drive (something like a car with a sputtering engine that can only keep up speed when the accelerator is pushed to the floor). The neurohumoral drive is characterized by high levels of renin, angiotensin II, aldosterone, catecholamines, and ADH. These signals stimulate the heart and cause the kidneys to retain sodium and water, which in principle should assist the heart by raising filling pressures. However, the failing heart does not increase its output and the increased fluid volume leads to edema in the lungs, and later, edema in peripheral tissues, which is why this is called *congestive* heart failure. Because of the high fluid volume, atrial pressures sensed by the cardiopulmonary baroreceptors are high. The high atrial pressures should lead to decreased ADH secretion and decreased sympathetic drive to the kidneys.[4] Instead, sympathetic activity and ADH are increased, and the kidneys operate at a new set-point in which normal sodium and water excretion occur only when there is excessive body fluid volume. Furthermore, the plasma concentration of sodium actually falls, producing hyponatremia, because water retention exceeds sodium retention. If fluid volume is somehow restored to normal levels, renal excretion of sodium drops to very low levels. Another characteristic of congestive heart failure is high levels of natriuretic peptides. This is an appropriate response to the high atrial pressures and partially counteracts the sodium-retaining actions of the kidneys, but does not restore sodium output to a level that would occur in a healthy person who transiently developed a high fluid volume (a volume that exists chronically in the heart failure patient). The high fluid volume of congestive heart failure is deleterious to pulmonary function and over time often leads to structural changes in the heart (dilation) that only exacerbates the defective pumping. Therapy for congestive heart failure includes drugs that directly or indirectly interfere with sodium-retaining processes in the kidneys. Diuretics directly increase sodium excretion. Drugs that inhibit the generation of angiotensin II (ACE inhibitors) or block the actions of angiotensin II (angiotensin receptor antagonists) reduce the signals that cause sodium retention.

Hypertension is both more common than congestive heart failure, and more difficult to understand. In some cases, the reason for the elevated blood pressure is clear. For example, renal glomerular disease often leads to inappropriate release of renin with subsequent increases in angiotensin II, aldosterone, collecting-tubule sodium reabsorption, and finally an increase in blood pressure. A tumor of the adrenal cortex can lead to excess production of aldosterone and increases in blood pressure; or a specific gain of function mutation in the sodium reabsorptive mechanism in the collecting duct also leads to excess sodium reabsorption and profound hypertension. These are all examples of secondary hypertension, that is, hypertension secondary to a known cause, whereas the vast majority of cases are called primary or essential hypertension, in which the cause is unknown. Research indicates that the intrarenal RAS is activated in essential hypertension, but there is debate whether this is the root of the problem or the result of inappropriate sympathetic stimulation. It is interesting that, unlike congestive heart failure, essential hypertension is not characterized by obvious signs of sodium retention such as swelling of the feet. However, current therapy employs most of the same drugs used to induce sodium loss, that is, diuretics, ACE inhibitors, AII receptor blockers, and aldosterone receptor blockers. At first glance this may seem paradoxical, because it is natural to ascribe the effectiveness of these agents to their reduction of sodium retention. But we remind the reader that the RAAS system has direct vascular actions, and inhibition of changes in peripheral resistance and vascular stiffness may account for most of their value. In addition, many drugs exhibit beneficial effects that cannot be accounted for on the basis of their known mechanisms of action, or the drugs are effective only with prolonged use.

KEY CONCEPTS

Sodium and water excretion are regulated primarily to meet the needs of the cardiovascular system via preservation of vascular volume and plasma osmolality.

The macula densa blunts changes in GFR via tubuloglomerular feedback.

Extracellular volume varies directly with sodium content.

Baroreceptors at various sites inform the kidneys of vascular pressures and volume status.

The renin-angiotensin system is the major controller of sodium excretion

Angiotensin II, produced by local and systemic renin-angiotensin systems, is a crucial regulator of sodium excretion and blood pressure via its actions in the kidneys, peripheral vasculature, and adrenal glands.

Aldosterone (in the presence of AII) stimulates sodium reabsorption by NCC in DCT cells and by ENaC in principal cells in the distal nephron.

Sympathetic stimulation is a major controller of sodium excretion.

Intrarenal dopamine plus several other mediators limit sodium reabsorption (increase excretion).

Water excretion varies in proportion to solute excretion and inversely with urine osmolality.

ADH secretion is regulated by plasma osmolality via osmoreceptors in the circum-ventricular organs, and by blood pressure via the baroreceptor-vasomotor center system.

Most cases of heart failure and hypertension involve hyperactivation of the RAAS and are commonly treated with drugs that block components of the RAAS.

STUDY QUESTIONS

7–1. Which of the following cell types are not nerve cells?

a. Pituitary cells that secrete ADH

b. Baroreceptors located in pulmonary vessels

c. Baroreceptors located in the arch of the aorta

d. Intrarenal baroreceptors

7–2. In the production of aldosterone, the rate-limiting step is:

a. the production of angiotensin I.

b. the production of angiotensinogen.

c. the activity of angiotensin-converting enzyme.

d. the responsiveness of the adrenal gland to angiotensin II.

7–3. A person eats a large bag of very salty potato chips with no beverage. Which response is most likely to ensue?

a. Movement of aquaporins into the apical membrane of cortical collecting duct principal cells.

b. Enhanced activity of Na-H antiporters in the proximal tubule.

c. Enhanced activity of Na-K-ATPase pumps in collecting duct principal cells.

d. Decreased levels of natriuretic peptides in the blood.

7–4. In response to a major hemorrhage:

a. The afferent arteriole vasodilates.

b. ADH secretion is reduced.

c. Granular (juxtaglomerular) cells are stimulated by neural input.

d. Neural baroreceptor firing rate increases.

7–5. The macula densa generates signals that directly regulate
   a. smooth muscle in afferent arterioles.
   b. tubular water permeability.
   c. ADH secretion.
   d. all of these.

7–6. Which one of the following will decrease sodium excretion?
   a. Decreased activity in the renal sympathetic nerve.
   b. Decreased levels of dopamine in the kidneys.
   c. Decreased levels of AII in the kidneys.
   d. Decreased levels of ADH in the kidneys.

Regulation of Potassium Balance

8

REGULATION OF POTASSIUM BETWEEN THE INTRACELLULAR AND EXTRACELLULAR COMPARTMENTS

The vast majority of body potassium is freely dissolved in the cytosol of tissue cells and constitutes the major osmotic component of the intracellular fluid (ICF). Only about 2% of total-body potassium is in the extracellular fluid (ECF). This small fraction, however, is absolutely crucial for body function, and the concentration of potassium in the ECF is a closely regulated quantity. Major increases and decreases (called hyperkalemia and hypokalemia) in

133

plasma values are cause for medical intervention. The importance of maintaining this concentration stems primarily from the role of potassium in the excitability of nerve and muscle, especially the heart. The ratio of the intracellular to extracellular concentration of potassium is the major determinant of the resting membrane potential in these cells. A significant rise in the extracellular potassium concentration causes a sustained depolarization. Low extracellular potassium may hyperpolarize or depolarize depending on how changes in extracellular potassium affect membrane permeability. Both conditions lead to muscle and cardiac disturbances.

> *The vast majority of body potassium is contained in tissue cells; only about 2% is in the ECF.*

Given that the vast majority of body potassium is contained within cells, the extracellular potassium concentration is crucially dependent on (1) the total amount of potassium in the body and (2) the *distribution* of this potassium between the ECF and ICF compartments. Total-body potassium is determined by the balance between potassium intake and excretion. Healthy individuals remain in potassium balance, as they do in sodium balance, by excreting potassium in response to dietary loads and reducing excretion when body potassium is depleted. The urine is the major route of potassium excretion, although some is lost in the feces and sweat. Normally the losses via sweat and the gastrointestinal tract are small, but large quantities can be lost from the digestive tract during diarrhea or severe vomiting. The control of renal potassium transport is the major mechanism by which total-body potassium is maintained in balance.

The fact that most body potassium is in the ICF follows strictly from the size and properties of the intracellular and extracellular compartments. About two-thirds of the body fluids are in the ICF, and typical cytosolic potassium concentrations are about 140 to 150 mEq/L. One-third of the body fluids are in the ECF, with a potassium concentration of about 4 mEq/L. In a clinical setting, only the extracellular concentration can be measured (the intracellular potassium is, in a sense, hidden behind the wall of the cell membrane). Furthermore, the extracellular value does not necessarily reflect total-body potassium. A patient may, for example, be hyperkalemic (high plasma potassium concentration) and yet at the same time be depleted of total-body potassium.

The high level of potassium within cells is maintained by the collective operation of the Na-K-ATPase plasma membrane pumps, which actively transport potassium into cells. Because the total amount of potassium in the extracellular compartment is so small (40–60 mEq total), even very slight shifts of potassium into or out of cells produce large changes in extracellular potassium concentration. Similarly, a meal rich in potassium (e.g., steak, potato, and spinach) could easily double the extracellular concentration of potassium if most of that potassium were not rapidly transferred from the blood to the intracellular compartment. It is crucial, therefore, that dietary loads be taken up into the intracellular compartment rapidly to prevent major changes in plasma potassium concentration.

The tissue contributing most to the sequestration of potassium is skeletal muscle, simply because muscle cells collectively contain the largest intracellular volume. Muscle effectively buffers extracellular potassium by taking up or releasing it to keep the plasma potassium concentration close to normal. On a moment-to-moment basis, this is what protects the ECF from large swings in potassium concentration. Major factors involved in these homeostatic processes include insulin and epinephrine, both of which cause increased potassium uptake by muscle and certain other cells through stimulation of plasma membrane Na-K-ATPases. Another influence is the GI tract, which contains an elaborate neural network (the "gut brain") that sends signals to the central nervous system. It also contains a complement of enteroendocrine cells that release an array of peptide hormones. Together these neural and hormonal signals affect many target organs, including the kidneys (see later discussion) in response to dietary input.

The increase in plasma insulin concentration after a meal is a crucial factor in moving potassium absorbed from the GI tract into cells rather than allowing it to accumulate in the ECF. This newly ingested potassium then slowly comes out of cells between meals to be excreted in the urine. Moreover, a large increase in plasma potassium concentration facilitates insulin secretion at any time, and the additional insulin induces greater potassium uptake by the cells, a negative feedback system for opposing acute elevations in plasma potassium concentration. In the natural order of things, insulin also stimulates glucose uptake and metabolism by cells: a necessary source of energy to drive the insulin-activated Na-K-ATPase responsible for moving potassium into cells.

On a moment-to-moment basis, plasma potassium is regulated by taking up or releasing potassium from tissue cells, primarily muscle.

The effect of epinephrine on cellular potassium uptake is probably of greatest physiological importance during exercise when potassium moves out of muscle cells that are rapidly firing action potentials. In fact, very intense intermittent exercise like wind sprints can actually double plasma potassium for a brief period. However, at the same time, exercise increases adrenal secretion of epinephrine, which stimulates potassium uptake by the Na-K-ATPase in muscle and other cells, and the transiently high potassium levels are restored to normal with a few minutes of rest.[1] Similarly, trauma causes loss of potassium from damaged cells, and epinephrine released due to stress stimulates other cells to take up plasma potassium.

Still another influence on the distribution of potassium between the ICF and ECF is the ECF hydrogen ion concentration: An increase in ECF hydrogen ion concentration (acidemia; see Chapter 9) is often associated with net potassium movement out of cells, whereas a decrease in ECF hydrogen ion concentration (alkalemia) causes net potassium movement into them. It is as though potassium

---

[1] Intense activity of the Na-K-ATPase hyperpolarizes the cells and prevents what otherwise would be a dangerous depolarization due to the high extracellular potassium.

and hydrogen ions were exchanging across plasma membranes (i.e., hydrogen ions moving into the cell during acidemia and out during alkalemia and potassium doing just the opposite), but the precise mechanism underlying these "exchanges" is not completely clear. However, like the effect of insulin, it probably involves an inhibition (acidemia) or activation (alkalemia) of the Na-K-ATPase.

RENAL POTASSIUM HANDLING

Overview

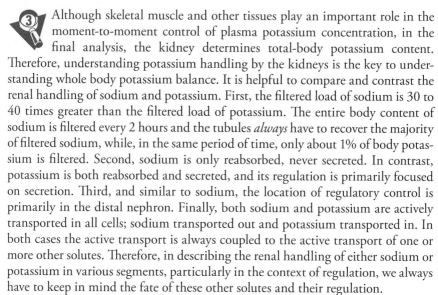 Although skeletal muscle and other tissues play an important role in the moment-to-moment control of plasma potassium concentration, in the final analysis, the kidney determines total-body potassium content. Therefore, understanding potassium handling by the kidneys is the key to understanding whole body potassium balance. It is helpful to compare and contrast the renal handling of sodium and potassium. First, the filtered load of sodium is 30 to 40 times greater than the filtered load of potassium. The entire body content of sodium is filtered every 2 hours and the tubules *always* have to recover the majority of filtered sodium, while, in the same period of time, only about 1% of body potassium is filtered. Second, sodium is only reabsorbed, never secreted. In contrast, potassium is both reabsorbed and secreted, and its regulation is primarily focused on secretion. Third, and similar to sodium, the location of regulatory control is primarily in the distal nephron. Finally, both sodium and potassium are actively transported in all cells; sodium transported out and potassium transported in. In both cases the active transport is always coupled to the active transport of one or more other solutes. Therefore, in describing the renal handling of either sodium or potassium in various segments, particularly in the context of regulation, we always have to keep in mind the fate of these other solutes and their regulation.

Potassium is freely filtered into Bowman's space, with a concentration identical to that in plasma, that is, ~4 mEq/L. Under all conditions, almost all the filtered load (~90%) is reabsorbed by the proximal tubule and thick ascending limb of the loop of Henle. Then, if the body is conserving potassium, most of the rest is reabsorbed in the distal nephron and medullary collecting ducts, leaving almost none in the urine. In contrast, if the body is ridding itself of potassium, which is the normal state of affairs, a large amount is secreted in the distal nephron, resulting in a substantial excretion. When secretion occurs at high rates, the amount excreted may even exceed the filtered load. The chief means of regulation lies in control of secretion in parts of the nephron beyond the loop of Henle. Let us look at potassium handling by various nephron segments and then address the issue of control.

Given that potassium is freely filtered, a normal plasma level of 4 mEq/L and GFR of 150 L/day or more results in a daily filtered load of about 600 mEq/day. The subsequent events in various tubule segments are summarized in Table 8–1. In the proximal tubule about 65% of the filtered load is reabsorbed, mostly via the paracellular route. The flux is driven by the increase in tubular concentration that occurs when water is reabsorbed, which, as we emphasized earlier, concentrates all solutes that have not been previously reabsorbed. This flux is essentially

Table 8–1. Percentage of filtered load transported at different locations depending on diet

Transport	Normal-or high-potassium diet	Low-potassium diet or potassium depletion
Proximal tubule	Reabsorption (65%)	Reabsorption (65%)
Thick ascending limb	Reabsorption (25%)	Reabsorption (25%)
Distal tubule and principal cells in the connecting tubule and cortical collecting duct	Secretion (20%–150%)	Little secretion
Intercalated cells, cortical collecting duct	Secretion (0%–5 %)	Reabsorption (5%)
Intercalated cells, medullary collecting duct	Reabsorption (5%)	Reabsorption (3%)
Final urine	20%–150%	2%

unregulated and varies mostly with how much sodium, and therefore water, is reabsorbed.

The proximal tubule pumping by the Na-K-ATPase is very vigorous, meaning there is a high rate of potassium uptake from the interstitium into the tubular cells. Since we know there is net potassium transport *to* the interstitium, this pumped potassium must therefore recycle right back by passive flux through channels in the basolateral membrane.

> *Almost all filtered potassium is reabsorbed. The amount excreted is controlled by how much is* **secreted**.

The loop of Henle continues the reabsorption of potassium. The major events take place in the thick ascending limb, where the Na-K-2Cl multiporter in the apical membrane of the tubular cells takes up potassium (see Figure 6–4). This is an active process driven by the electrochemical gradient for sodium. The tubule contains far less potassium than sodium, but the Na-K-2Cl transporter moves equal amounts of each one. Therefore, to supply enough potassium to accompany the large amount of sodium being reabsorbed by the symporter, potassium must recycle back to the lumen by passive flux through channels. If this did not happen then sodium reabsorption would be limited only to the amount of potassium present in the tubular fluid.

Not all of the potassium entering from the lumen recycles back to the lumen; some moves through the cells and exits across the basolateral membrane, thereby constituting a net potassium reabsorption. There is additional potassium entering from the interstitium via the Na-K-ATPase, similar to the situation in the proximal tubule, and it also exits back to the interstitium. Cellular potassium moving into the interstitium leaves by a combination of passive flux through channels and flux through K-Cl symporters with chloride. Some potassium is also reabsorbed by the paracellular route in this segment, driven by a lumen-positive voltage. The sum of these transcellular and paracellular processes is net potassium reabsorption of about 25% of the filtered load. Combined with the 65% previously reabsorbed in the proximal tubule, only about 10% is passed on to the distal nephron.

At this point the process becomes more complicated, as the distal nephron expresses both reabsorptive and secretory mechanisms. It is the quantitative activity of each that determines net potassium excretion. This flexibility requires the existence of several types of transporters and channels whose activity can be varied up or down to yield an appropriate final level of excretion. Because of the many components in this process let us first identify the major transport elements and their location before explaining how they are controlled.

As described earlier (see Chapter 6), the distal nephron is composed of a several segments. The distal convoluted tubule is usually divided into two parts with morphologically different cell types. The cells of the late distal tubule contain the type of potassium channels known as ROMK (standing for *renal outer medulla potassium (K)* channel, because that is where they were first identified). These cells secrete potassium at rates that vary with conditions. The connecting tubule and the cortical collecting tubule contain principal cells (about 70% of the cells) interspersed with intercalated cells. The principal cells also contain ROMK channels that secrete potassium at variable rates. This rate depends on the simultaneous uptake of sodium via ENaC channels where there is, in effect, a functional exchange of reabsorbed sodium for secreted potassium (Figure 8–1). The intercalated cells are further subdivided into type A (more numerous), type B (sparse), and a third type called non-A non-B cells. The differences between the various types of intercalated cells are crucial for the renal handling of acids and bases and will be covered more thoroughly in Chapter 9. Type A intercalated cells have mechanisms for both secretion and reabsorption of potassium. When reabsorbing, the normal case, they take up potassium from the tubule via an H-K antiporter that simultaneously secretes a proton. The potassium is released into the interstitium via a basolateral channel (Figure 8–2). The type A intercalated cells also express a potassium channel called *BK* (since each channel has a "big" capacity to secrete potassium; also called maxi-K channels). Normally these channels are closed, but under conditions of high potassium excretion the type A cells take up potassium from the interstitium via an Na-K-2Cl multiporter in the basolateral membrane and secrete potassium via the BK channels in the apical membrane.

All of the above endows the nephron with a great flexibility to deal with a wide range of dietary input (see Figure 8–3). Finally, the *medullary* collecting ducts reabsorb small amounts of potassium under all conditions. When the sum of upstream processes has already reabsorbed almost all the potassium, the medullary collecting ducts bring the final urine excretion down to a few percent of the filtered load, for an excretion of about 10 to 15 mEq/day (compared to a filtration rate of ~600 mEq/day). On the other hand, if upstream segments are secreting avidly, the modest reabsorption in the medullary collecting ducts does little to alter an excretion that can reach 1000 mEq/day. Figure 8–4 depicts the overall renal handling of potassium in different tubule regions in conditions of high and low potassium excretion.

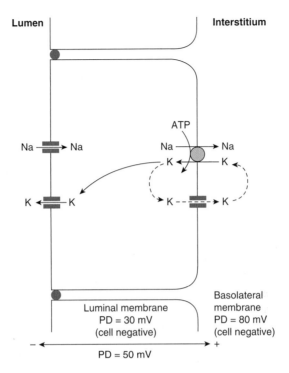

Figure 8–1. Generalized pathway for potassium secretion by principal cells. Potassium secretion is increased by sodium entry through ENaC sodium channels because (1) this stimulates the Na-K-ATPase and (2) depolarizes the luminal membrane. Potassium entering via the Na-K-ATPase that is not secreted recycles through basolateral channels.

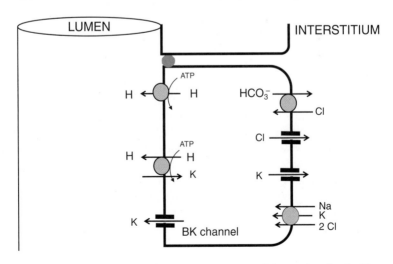

Figure 8–2. Transport pathways for potassium in type A intercalated cells. These cells reabsorb potassium and secrete hydrogen ions via H-K-ATPases and H-ATPases as shown in the upper part of the figure. In response to large potassium loads the secretory pathway for potassium via BK channels shown in the bottom of the figure becomes active.

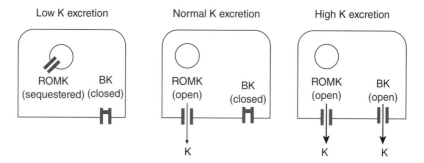

Figure 8–3. Activity of ROMK and BK potassium channels under different conditions. When the body is conserving potassium and little is being excreted, ROMK channels are mostly sequestered in intracellular vesicles and BK channels are closed; thus there is virtually no secretion. Under modest potassium loads (normal conditions), ROMK channels secrete potassium, while BK channels remain closed. When potassium excretion is very high, as on a high-potassium diet, ROMK channel activity is maximized and BK channels are open, allowing substantial secretion.

CONTROL OF POTASSIUM EXCRETION

The regulation of potassium excretion is as complicated as the regulation of sodium excretion. It is particularly noteworthy that, as noted earlier, potassium transport mechanisms in the distal nephron are always coupled to the transport of other substances, chiefly sodium and hydrogen, yet under normal circumstances variations in the excretion of these other substances does not prevent the kidneys from appropriately excreting potassium.[2] We emphasize normal because there are many pathological conditions in which this independence is compromised. In the following paragraphs, we list several known regulatory factors (see Figure 8–5).

Dietary Potassium

It goes without saying that the overall determinant of renal potassium excretion is dietary input. But how the kidneys "know" about dietary input is still somewhat mysterious. While very large potassium loads can increase plasma potassium somewhat, the changes in excretion associated with ordinary fluctuations in dietary input do not seem to be accounted for on the basis of either changes in plasma potassium or other identified factors. One factor known to exert an influence, but not the major one, is the previously mentioned gastrointestinal peptide hormones released in response to ingested potassium. These hormones not only influence the cellular uptake of potassium absorbed from the GI tract, but also the renal handling of potassium, and seem to be one of the links between dietary load and excretion.

---

[2]Large loads of sodium or potassium cause transient increases in the excretion of the other, but over time proper balance is reestablished for each one.

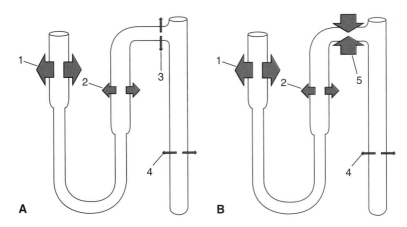

Figure 8–4. Potassium transport in conditions of high or low excretion. **A,** When potassium excretion is low, the majority of filtered potassium is reabsorbed in the proximal tubule, mainly by the paracellular route (1). In the thick ascending limb most of the rest is reabsorbed, mostly by the transcellular route (2). In the cortical (3) and medullary collecting duct (4) there is some additional reabsorption via intercalated cells. **B,** When potassium excretion is high the events in most regions of the tubule are the same as when there is little potassium excretion, but in the distal nephron there is major secretion (5) that in some cases is greater than the sum of the reabsorptive processes.

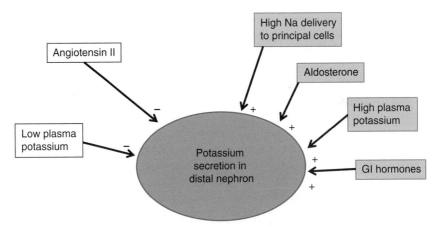

Figure 8–5. Factors that influence secretion of potassium as described in the text.

A manifestation of changing dietary loads over time is to regulate the distribution of ROMK channels between the apical membrane and intracellular storage, that is, high-potassium diets lead to insertion of apical channels and therefore higher potassium secretion. In contrast, during periods of prolonged low potassium ingestion, there are few ROMK channels in the apical membrane. Yet another adaptation to prolonged periods of low potassium ingestion is an increase in H-K-ATPase activity in intercalated cells, resulting in even more efficient reabsorption of filtered potassium.

Plasma Potassium

 Plasma potassium, when it deviates from normal, is an understandable influence. First, the filtered load is directly proportional to plasma concentration. Second, the environment of the cells that secrete potassium, that is, the cortical interstitium, has a potassium concentration that is nearly the same as in plasma. The Na-K-ATPase that takes up potassium in principal cells is highly sensitive to the potassium concentration in this space, and varies its pump rate up and down when potassium levels in the plasma vary up and down. Also, high potassium levels shift sodium reabsorption from distal tubule cells to cortical tubule cells with a concomitant increase in distal tubule potassium secretion. The delivery of additional fluid and potassium to the collecting tubule stimulates potassium secretion (see further explanation below). Thus, plasma potassium concentration exerts an influence on potassium excretion, but is not the dominant factor under normal conditions.

Aldosterone

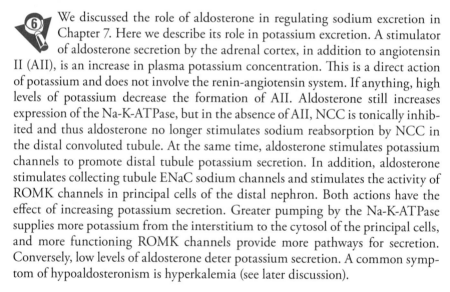 We discussed the role of aldosterone in regulating sodium excretion in Chapter 7. Here we describe its role in potassium excretion. A stimulator of aldosterone secretion by the adrenal cortex, in addition to angiotensin II (AII), is an increase in plasma potassium concentration. This is a direct action of potassium and does not involve the renin-angiotensin system. If anything, high levels of potassium decrease the formation of AII. Aldosterone still increases expression of the Na-K-ATPase, but in the absence of AII, NCC is tonically inhibited and thus aldosterone no longer stimulates sodium reabsorption by NCC in the distal convoluted tubule. At the same time, aldosterone stimulates potassium channels to promote distal tubule potassium secretion. In addition, aldosterone stimulates collecting tubule ENaC sodium channels and stimulates the activity of ROMK channels in principal cells of the distal nephron. Both actions have the effect of increasing potassium secretion. Greater pumping by the Na-K-ATPase supplies more potassium from the interstitium to the cytosol of the principal cells, and more functioning ROMK channels provide more pathways for secretion. Conversely, low levels of aldosterone deter potassium secretion. A common symptom of hypoaldosteronism is hyperkalemia (see later discussion).

Angiotensin II

AII is an *inhibitor* of potassium secretion. Its mechanism of action is to decrease the activity of ROMK channels in principal cells, thereby limiting the potassium flux from cell to lumen. Thus, AII and aldosterone exert influences on potassium excretion in opposite directions (unlike their concerted action to promote sodium reabsorption).

A key determinant of potassium secretion is sodium delivery to principal cells beyond the distal tubule.

Sodium Delivery to the Distal Nephron

Sodium delivery to cells in the connecting tubule and cortical collecting duct is a major regulator of potassium secretion. High sodium delivery stimulates potassium secretion; low sodium delivery inhibits it. The influence is exerted on both principal and intercalated cells. In principal cells, sodium entry via sodium channels depolarizes the apical membrane and thereby increases the electrochemical gradient driving the outward flow of potassium through channels (similar in principle to what happens during action potentials in excitable cells). Second, more sodium delivered means more sodium taken up and pumped out by the Na-K-ATPase, in turn causing more potassium to be pumped in. In conditions of high sodium delivery, the BK channels in type A intercalated cells also play a role. They become activated and secrete potassium in parallel with ROMK channels in principal cells. The signaling pathway is not fully understood, but may involve flow sensing by apical cilia, similar to what happens in macula densa cells. Because potassium secretion in the distal nephron is strongly influenced by sodium delivery, the amount secreted is, therefore, strongly affected by the amount of sodium reabsorbed in prior segments (see below).

1. Only a small fraction of body potassium is in the ECF, and the extracellular concentration may not be a good indicator of total-body potassium status.
2. On a short-term basis, uptake and release of potassium by tissue cells prevent large swings in extracellular potassium concentration.
3. Overall renal handling is accomplished by reabsorbing nearly all filtered potassium and then secreting an amount of potassium that maintains balance between ingestion and excretion.
4. It is mainly the principal cells of the connecting tubule and cortical collecting duct that alter rates of potassium secretion.
5. Potassium secretion (and thus excretion) is increased by high sodium delivery to the distal nephron, particularly when this is caused by diuretics acting upstream.

Simultaneous Regulation of Sodium and Potassium

Sodium and potassium loads vary over time, sometimes in parallel and sometimes in opposite directions. The healthy body is able to excrete or withhold excretion of each one independently (recognizing that major changes in dietary loads of one have transient effects on the excretion of the other). Part of the ability of the body to adapt to dietary changes resides in altered expression of relevant transport proteins. However, a major signal that controls the excretion of both sodium and potassium is aldosterone, which raises the question: how can one signal result in independent regulation of two variables? This question is often called the "*aldosterone paradox.*" It is resolved by recognizing the roles of AII, sodium delivery to principal cells, and the influence of potassium on aldosterone secretion (in the absence of AII). If most of the sodium leaving the loop of Henle is reabsorbed in the distal tubule, little remains to reach principal cells in the connecting tubule and collecting duct, and thus potassium secretion is not stimulated. In contrast, if modest or large amounts of sodium reach the principal cells, this results in considerable potassium secretion. Let us consider several examples of differing requirements for sodium and potassium excretion.

Case 1: Volume/sodium depletion with normal body potassium. The goal is to reabsorb as much sodium as possible while excreting potassium modestly. The volume/sodium depletion strongly activates the RAAS, generating high levels of both AII and aldosterone. The AII stimulates sodium reabsorption via Na-Cl symporters in the distal tubule. Consequently, relatively little sodium remains in the tubular fluid by the time it reaches the principal cells in the connecting tubule. Although those cells are being stimulated by aldosterone, and in theory, are capable of secreting large amounts of potassium, the relatively low amount of sodium available to be reabsorbed via ENaC channels limits the potential driving force for potassium at the apical membrane and how much sodium, and therefore potassium, can be transported by the Na-K-ATPase. Furthermore, AII specifically inhibits ROMK activity in principal cells. The end result is that sodium is saved without excessive loss of potassium.

Case 2: Potassium overload with normal ECF volume. The goal now is to increase potassium secretion without excessive reabsorption or excretion of sodium. AII levels are low (there is nothing to stimulate it), but aldosterone levels are high due to the high plasma potassium. Under these conditions, the lack of AII prevents aldosterone from stimulating NCC activity, but does allow aldosterone to stimulate potassium channels in the distal tubule.[3] Therefore, significant amounts of sodium bypass reabsorption in the distal tubule and instead are reabsorbed by principal cells. The limited sodium reabsorption in the distal tubule also leads to increased flow to the connecting tubule and collecting duct. Principal cells now reabsorb enough sodium via ENaCs, stimulated by aldosterone, to prevent excessive sodium loss. Simultaneously, the secretion of potassium occurs at a high rate from both principal and intercalated cells, stimulated by the increased flow and by aldosterone (without the inhibiting influence of AII). The combined result is high potassium excretion and normal sodium excretion. Figure 8–6 illustrates how high aldosterone, with or without simultaneous high AII, affects secretion of potassium.

Case 3: Depletion of both sodium and potassium. The goal is to maximize reabsorption of both sodium and potassium and excrete little of either one. The sodium depletion stimulates renin secretion and the production of AII, but the low potassium inhibits the ability of the adrenal glands to secrete aldosterone. Sodium is strongly reabsorbed in the distal tubule upstream from the principal cells, stimulated by AII,

---

[3] This effect is mediated by a complex signaling pathway dependent on membrane potential. Depolarization of distal tubule cells leads to the shutting down of a kinase that stimulates sodium reabsorption via the sodium-chloride symporter.

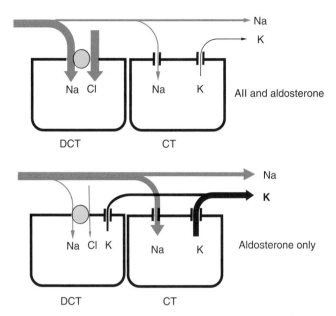

Figure 8–6. Difference in the effect of aldosterone on potassium secretion with and without angiotensin II. At the top, when the full RAAS system is activated by volume depletion, angiotensin II and aldosterone working together activate thiazide-sensitive NCC in the distal tubule to reabsorb substantial amounts of sodium. At the same, angiotensin II inhibits potassium secretory channels in the distal tubule. Aldosterone also stimulates ENaC in collecting tubule principal cells so that sodium that is not reabsorbed in the distal tubule can be reabsorbed in the collecting tubule with some concomitant low level of secretion of potassium through potassium channels in the cortical tubule cells. Levels of sodium and potassium in the final urine will be low. In the lower schematic, blood levels of potassium are high so aldosterone is elevated. However, there is little if any angiotensin II. Without angiotensin II, NCC in the distal tubule is inhibited and cannot be stimulated by aldosterone, but aldosterone does stimulate secretion from potassium channels. In the collecting tubule, aldosterone promotes uptake of sodium by ENaC in principal cells; a combination of aldosterone and increased flow strongly activate potassium channels in both principal cells and type A intercalated cells to secrete large amounts of potassium. Levels of sodium in the final urine will vary, but levels of potassium in the final urine will be high.

and principal cells are not stimulated by aldosterone. Since little potassium can be excreted without significant secretion, both sodium and potassium are reabsorbed.

There is yet another mechanism to allow control of potassium excretion independent of sodium that comes into play in cases of prolonged high dietary potassium and low dietary sodium, a condition faced by our distant ancestors. An adaptation to this condition is an increase in the activity of basolateral Na-H antiporters in principal cells. This supports the influx of sodium when the availability of sodium from the luminal side is very limited. Sodium entering via the Na-H antiporters is then removed by the Na-K-ATPase, that is, it is recycled. The continued operation of the Na-K-ATPase imports potassium, which is then secreted across the apical membrane. This adaptation allows the kidneys to excrete potassium while conserving sodium and underscores the remarkable ability of the kidneys to modify transporter abundance in order to preserve balance on a longer time scale.

Perturbations in Potassium Excretion: Diuretics

Up to this point we have emphasized the ability of the kidneys to regulate the excretion of sodium, potassium, and other substances independently and to handle any combination of loads. However, there are situations in which pathology, medical intervention, or excessive loss of one of these substances affects the excretion of another. We address this issue here and again in Chapter 9 in association with acid-base balance.

A common medical intervention is the use of diuretics. These are agents that increase urine flow, often called "water pills" by patients. The goal of diuretic use is to reduce ECF volume, thereby correcting or preventing edema. Diuretics work by increasing sodium excretion, which increases the osmotic load in the urine, taking water with it. Many diuretics, although effective at increasing water and sodium excretion, have the unwanted and serious side effect of increasing the renal excretion of potassium, leading to hypokalemia. The most powerful diuretics act by blocking sodium reabsorption by the Na-K-2Cl symporter in the thick ascending limb. These are called "loop diuretics" because they act in the loop of Henle. Another group, called thiazide diuretics, blocks the Na-Cl symporter in the distal tubule. Both classes of diuretic reduce sodium reabsorption upstream from the connecting tubule, and therefore result in a large amount of sodium delivered to downstream principal cells. This greatly stimulates sodium uptake in principal cells, but the high load overwhelms their transport capacity and most of it passes by and is excreted. The sodium that is reabsorbed in principal cells stimulates potassium secretion, leading to the unwanted hypokalemia. The potassium loss may cause severe potassium depletion (Figure 8–7).

Because potassium loss is so troubling, other classes of diuretics have been developed that are called "potassium-sparing." The drug amiloride blocks the ENaC sodium channels in principal cells, thereby obviating the stimulation of potassium secretion. Another class of diuretics blocks the renal actions of aldosterone. Such drugs are weak diuretics, but are also potassium-sparing because they block the stimulation of potassium channels by aldosterone that promotes potassium secretion.

A relatively new class of drugs, the vaptans, block vasopressin receptors. One, tolvaptan, blocks V_2 (ADH) receptors; therefore, they are useful to induce pure water loss with little or no sodium or potassium loss. The drug is useful for treating hyponatremia or congestive heart failure.

Perturbations in Potassium Excretion: Hyperkalemia

Hyperkalemia is a condition of elevated plasma potassium concentration (usually defined as potassium levels above 5.5 mEq/L). In principle, hyperkalemia can develop in two ways: (1) as a result of shifts of potassium from the ICF to the

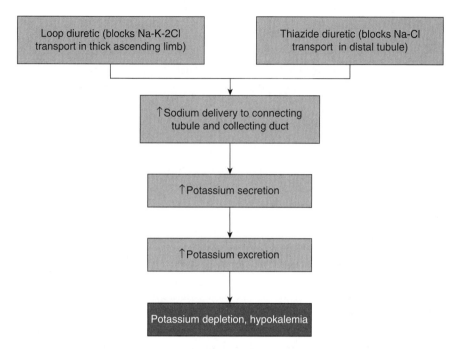

Figure 8–7. Pathways by which diuretic drugs affecting either the loop of Henle (loop diuretics) or distal convoluted tubule (thiazide diuretics) cause potassium depletion. Loop diuretics block potassium reabsorption in the thick ascending limb, but for both classes of diuretic the major factor leading to increased potassium excretion is increased delivery of sodium to principal cells and increased luminal flow in the distal nephron, both of which stimulate potassium secretion.

ECF or (2) from an increase in total-body potassium. Shifts can be induced by an increase in plasma hydrogen ion concentration, as occurs during a metabolic acidosis (see Chapter 9), and occurs transiently during intense exercise as described earlier. Most cases of *chronic* hyperkalemia are a result of whole body potassium overload and involve inability of the kidneys to excrete potassium adequately.

An obvious renal cause of hyperkalemia is chronic renal failure. In terms of excretion, the kidneys can compensate for reduced GFR to a considerable extent (e.g., we can get by well with just one kidney), but when GFR falls to only 10% of normal, hyperkalemia is a likely consequence. The reason is simply that the kidneys have lost potassium transport capacity. Because chronic hyperkalemia is life threatening, renal dialysis or transplant becomes necessary.

Another pathology leading to hyperkalemia is *hypoaldosteronism*. This condition can itself be the result of several causes, including primary adrenal insufficiency (the adrenal gland cannot synthesize aldosterone) and hyporeninemic hypoaldosteronism, which is failure to secrete enough renin. The result either way is that plasma levels of aldosterone are abnormally low, and the actions of aldosterone to stimulate potassium secretion are severely decreased. A variant of this condition is pseudohypoaldosteronism, in which the principal cells do not respond to aldosterone. Again the result is decreased capacity to secrete, and therefore to excrete potassium.

Another common cause of hyperkalemia is medical intervention. Just as powerful diuretics often lead to *hypo*kalemia, some treatments for cardiac failure often lead to *hyper*kalemia. Common treatments for cardiac failure involve concomitant use of ACE inhibitors (block production of AII) and potassium-sparing diuretics. The combination prevents sufficient action of aldosterone in renal principal cells, again leading to decreased potassium secretion.

KEY CONCEPTS

 Potassium is distributed predominantly in the intracellular compartment, and the extracellular concentration may not be a good indicator of total-body potassium status.

 On a short-term basis, uptake and release of potassium by muscle stabilizes extracellular potassium concentration.

 Almost all filtered potassium is reabsorbed, with secretion by distal convoluted tubule and cortical tubule cells in the distal nephron determining the amount excreted.

 The rate of potassium secretion is set by active influx across the basolateral membrane and apical channel activity.

 Potassium secretion (and thus excretion) is increased by high sodium delivery to the distal nephron, particularly when this is caused by diuretics acting upstream.

 AII with aldosterone inhibits potassium secretion; aldosterone in the absence of AII stimulates potassium secretion.

STUDY QUESTIONS

8–1. Potassium excretion is controlled mainly by controlling the rate of:
   a. potassium reabsorption in the proximal tubule.
   b. potassium reabsorption in the distal nephron.
   c. potassium secretion in the proximal tubule.
   d. potassium secretion in the distal nephron.

8–2. In the thick ascending limb:

    a. the net amounts of potassium and sodium that are reabsorbed are about the same.

    b. the major pathway for moving potassium from lumen to cell is via the Na-K-ATPase.

    c. most of the potassium that is reabsorbed into the cells leaks back into the lumen via potassium channels.

    d. the major pathway for moving potassium from cell to interstitium is via the Na-K-2Cl multiporter.

8–3. For which substance is it possible to excrete more than is filtered?

    a. Sodium

    b. Potassium

    c. Chloride

    d. It is not possible to excrete any of these ions in amounts greater than the filtered loads.

8–4. After a potassium-rich meal, the key action of insulin that prevents a large increase in plasma potassium is to:

    a. decrease absorption of potassium from the GI tract.

    b. increase uptake of potassium by tissue cells.

    c. increase the filtered load of potassium.

    d. increase tubular secretion of potassium.

8–5. A key role of "BK" potassium channels in the kidney is to

    a. reabsorb potassium when the body is depleted of potassium.

    b. recycle potassium in the thick ascending limb.

    c. secrete potassium when distal nephron flow rate is very low.

    d. help the body excrete potassium in response to very large loads.

8–6. Which of the following has the effect of reducing the excretion of potassium?

    a. The actions of angiotensin II on the kidney.

    b. The actions of aldosterone on the kidney.

    c. Decreased sodium reabsorption in the loop of Henle.

    d. Activation of BK channels in principal cells.

Regulation of Acid-Base Balance

9

OBJECTIVES

▶ State the Henderson-Hasselbalch equation for the carbon dioxide-bicarbonate buffer system.

▶ State the major sources for the input of fixed acids and bases into the body, including metabolic processes and activities of the gastrointestinal tract.

▶ Describe how the input of fixed acids and bases affects body levels of bicarbonate.

▶ Explain why body levels of carbon dioxide are usually not altered by the input of fixed acids and bases.

▶ Explain why some low pH fluids alkalinize the blood after they are metabolized.

▶ Describe the reabsorption of filtered bicarbonate by the proximal tubule.

▶ Describe how bicarbonate is excreted in response to an alkaline load.

▶ Describe how excretion of acid and generation of new bicarbonate are linked.

▶ Describe how the titration of filtered bases is a means of excreting acid.

▶ Describe how the conversion of glutamine to ammonium and subsequent excretion of ammonium accomplishes the goal of excreting acid.

▶ Describe how the kidneys handle ammonium that has been secreted in the proximal tubule.

▶ State how total acid excretion is related to titratable acidity and ammonium excretion.

▶ Define the four categories of primary acid-base disturbance and the meaning of compensation.

▶ Describe the renal response to respiratory acid-base disorders.

▶ Identify the primary types of renal tubular acidosis (RTA).

OVERVIEW

A key task of the body is to regulate acid-base balance. Perturbations in acid-base balance are among the most important problems confronting clinicians in a hospital setting. The kidneys are major players in the excretion of acids and bases and in the maintenance of acid-base balance. As explained below, the kidneys work in partnership with other organ systems, primarily the respiratory system and the liver to keep plasma acid-base status within normal limits.

It is essential for the body to control the concentration of free protons (hydrogen ions) in the ECF. While most substances regulated by renal processes exist at concentrations in the millimolar range or greater, the normal hydrogen ion concentration is a seemingly miniscule 40 nanomolar (one nanomole is *one millionth* of a millimole). Even though very small, this level is crucial for body function. Proteins contain titratable groups that reversibly bind hydrogen ions. As sites on membrane proteins protonate and deprotonate in response to changes in extracellular pH, the resulting alteration of local charge density affects the shape, and therefore the behavior of those proteins. The plasma levels of hydrogen ions are constantly being altered by a number of processes, including (1) metabolism of ingested food, (2) secretions of the gastrointestinal (GI) tract, (3) de novo generation of acids and bases from metabolism of stored fat and glycogen, and (4) changes in the production of carbon dioxide.

The essence of the physiological response to these changes comes down to two processes: (1) match the *excretion* of acid-base equivalents to their input, that is, maintain balance and (2) regulate the *ratio* of weak acids to their conjugate bases in buffer systems. Buffer systems limit changes in pH to a small range. The two processes of excreting acids and bases, and regulating physiological buffer concentrations are intimately related, but they are not identical. It is possible to be in balance even though buffer ratios are inappropriate.

ACID-BASE FUNDAMENTALS

Acid-base physiology differs from that of the other substances discussed earlier in the text in a fundamental way. Mineral ions and organic solutes such as urea exist in the body as independent entities. We can describe the concentration of any one of these substances without reference to any others. Acid-base physiology is different. It always involves a set of three interacting substances: an acid, a base, and a hydrogen ion (proton). The existence of one implies the existence of the other two, and changes in one always bring about changes in the other two. As shown in Equation 9-1, when acids are dissolved in water they dissociate into a hydrogen ion and a conjugate base. Analogously, a base dissolved in water combines with existing hydrogen ions to form an acid.[1] Regardless of the starting materials, the three substances will come to equilibrium with a fixed relationship as shown in Equation 9-2, where K is the dissociation constant. Strong acids such as hydrochloric acid fully dissociate and release all their hydrogen ions when dissolved in water. For example, if we dissolve 1 mmol of hydrochloric acid, we produce 1 mmol of free hydrogen ions. On the other hand, weak acids like acetic acid or lactic acid keep most of the hydrogen ions bound. If we dissolve 1 mmol of a weak

---

[1] A base is any substance that can bind a hydrogen ion (e.g., OH^-, lactate⁻). The term "conjugate base" means the particular base formed when a given acid dissociates a proton.

acid, the resulting number of free hydrogen ions is only a few percent of 1 mmol. Despite this small fraction, a weak acid present at a millimolar concentration in the blood would dissociate enough hydrogen ions to completely overwhelm the existing nanomolar level of free hydrogen ions if buffer systems did not intervene.

$$\text{acid} \leftrightharpoons \text{conjugate base} + H^+ \qquad\qquad \text{Equation 9-1}$$

$$[H^+] = K[\text{acid}]/[\text{base}] \qquad\qquad \text{Equation 9-2}$$

$$pH = pK + \log[\text{base/acid}] \qquad\qquad \text{Equation 9-3}$$

While the existence of an acid in solution always implies the existence of its conjugate base, if we place just weak acid in solution, there will only be miniscule amounts of the conjugate base because of limited dissociation. However, we can independently increase the conjugate base concentration by adding the salt of the acid. For example, if we mix acetic acid and potassium acetate there will be substantial levels of both the acid and the conjugate base. Such a mixture is a *buffer system*. A buffer system serves the useful purpose of limiting the change in pH upon addition of other acids or bases. When another acid is added, most of the hydrogen ions released by that acid combine with the conjugate base of the buffer system, greatly restricting the increase in free hydrogen ions. Similarly, when another base is added, most of the free hydrogen ions that combine with the base are replaced by hydrogen ions that dissociate from the acid of the buffer system.

In any buffer system, the *ratio* of the acid to its conjugate base fixes the free aqueous concentration of hydrogen ion (which is only a trivial fraction of the concentration of either the acid or base), as shown in Equation 9-2, or in the more familiar pH form (the Henderson-Hasselbalch equation) in Equation 9-3. We should emphasize that buffer systems in the body do not *eliminate* added acid or base equivalents, but only limit the effect of the equivalents on blood pH. In the face of persistent imbalance between acid-base input and output, one or the other component of the buffer is gradually reduced in concentration. Eventually acid or base equivalents added to the body, even though transiently associated with blood buffers, must be excreted by the kidneys to maintain balance.

Buffer systems exist in the extracellular fluid, the intracellular fluid (the cytosol of the various cells in the body), and in the matrix of bone. Although these buffers are in different compartments, they communicate with each other. Phosphate and albumin are important buffers in the ECF. Hemoglobin in red blood cells is an important intracellular buffer, since changes in plasma pH lead to uptake or release of protons from red blood cells. For several reasons, the most important buffer system in the body turns out to be the CO_2-*bicarbonate buffer system*. Fortunately, we can understand the role of buffers in acid-base balance by looking at this single buffer system alone and ignore the others, because all buffer systems are exposed to the same hydrogen ion concentration, and therefore must have ratios of weak acid to conjugate base that result in the same pH. This is known as the *isohydric principle*.

 One property that sets the CO_2-bicarbonate buffer system apart from other buffer systems is that the concentrations of CO_2 and bicarbonate are regulated independently. And because the concentrations of both components are regulated, the *ratio* of their concentrations is regulated. Therefore this regulates pH.

In the CO_2-bicarbonate buffer system, CO_2 is not a weak acid per se, but it is functionally a weak acid because it readily combines with water to form *carbonic acid* (H_2CO_3). Whenever a solution contains CO_2 it always contains a small amount of carbonic acid. (CO_2 is often called a volatile acid because it can evaporate. All other acids, for example, sulfuric, lactic, are called *fixed* acids.) Carbonic acid dissociates as does any other weak acid into a proton and its conjugate base, which is bicarbonate (Equation 9-4a). Considered this way, and given the ubiquitous presence of water in our body, it is clear that carbon dioxide is effectively an acid.

The concentration of carbonic acid in our blood is trivial (about 3 μmol/L), and at first glance it appears that this system has little buffering capacity. However, the supply of CO_2 is effectively infinite because it is being produced continuously (over 10 mol per day). Any carbonic acid consumed in a reaction is immediately replaced by new generation from existing CO_2 as shown in left half of Equation 9-4a.

$$CO_2 + H_2O \leftrightarrows H_2CO_3 \leftrightarrows HCO_3^- + H^+ \qquad \text{Equation 9-4a}$$

$$\underset{\text{(carbonic anhydrase)}}{CO_2 + H_2O \leftrightarrows HCO_3^- + H^+} \qquad \text{Equation 9-4b}$$

The reaction on the left side of Equation 9-4a to form carbonic acid is rather slow, but most tissues express one or several isoforms of the enzyme, *carbonic anhydrase*, intracellularly, extracellularly, or both. This enzyme greatly speeds the reaction between CO_2 and water to form bicarbonate and a hydrogen ion. In so doing it actually skips the step of forming carbonic acid, as shown in Equation 9-4b.[2] However, as with all enzyme-catalyzed reactions, the enzyme increases the *velocity* of the reaction but not the equilibrium concentrations of reactants and products.

Unlike the other buffer systems in the body, where addition or loss of hydrogen ions changes the concentration of the weak acid, in the CO_2-bicarbonate system, the concentration of the weak acid (CO_2) is held essentially constant. This is because the rate of respiratory excretion is matched to metabolic production. The partial pressure of arterial CO_2 (PCO_2) is regulated to be about 40 mm Hg. This partial pressure corresponds to a CO_2 concentration in blood of 1.2 mmol/L. Any change in PCO_2 resulting from the addition or loss of hydrogen ions or change in metabolic production is sensed by arterial chemoreceptors and chemoreceptors in the brainstem, which alter the rate of ventilation to restore the concentration. There are times when the PCO_2 does indeed differ from 40 mm Hg, but this reflects changes in the activity of the respiratory system, not a change in PCO_2 in response to addition or loss of hydrogen ions.

---

[2] The actual reaction involves combining CO_2 with a hydroxyl ion (OH^-) that is bound to the enzyme, resulting in the immediate formation of bicarbonate (HCO_3^-). As the bicarbonate dissociates from the enzyme, a water molecule replaces it. The water is then split into a hydrogen ion and a hydroxyl ion. The hydrogen ion dissociates from the enzyme and the hydroxyl ion stays behind on the enzyme. The end result is that a CO_2 molecule and a water molecule are converted to a hydrogen ion and bicarbonate, the same as if they had gone through the slower un-catalyzed reaction of first forming a carbonic acid molecule.

Although adding or removing hydrogen ions from a source other than CO_2 does not change PCO_2, such changes *do* change the concentration of bicarbonate. Adding hydrogen ions drives the reaction in Equations 9-4a and 9-4b to the left and reduces bicarbonate on a nearly mole-for-mole basis. We say nearly because the other blood buffers also take up some of the load. Removing hydrogen ions drives the reaction to the right and increases bicarbonate in the same way (see Figure 9–1). There are many processes that add or remove hydrogen ions, but regardless of the process, the result is to change the concentration of bicarbonate. This is a crucial concept, and therefore warrants re-emphasizing. From an acid-base perspective, any metabolic process or reaction that produces hydrogen ions is identical to one that removes bicarbonate (because in both cases the end result is loss of bicarbonate), and any reaction that consumes hydrogen ions is equivalent to one that produces bicarbonate (because in both cases the end result is an increase in bicarbonate).

From the foregoing we conclude that the task of maintaining hydrogen ion balance really becomes one of maintaining bicarbonate balance (again assuming that the respiratory system keeps PCO_2 constant) because the pH is set by the ratio of bicarbonate to PCO_2. When chemical reactions or cell activities alter the amount of bicarbonate in the blood, the body must either excrete the excess or replace the lost bicarbonate with new bicarbonate. Excretion and generation of new bicarbonate is the responsibility of the kidneys.

Before moving on, let us clarify a common misconception. At first glance it might seem that fixed acid equivalents could be converted to CO_2 and excreted by exhalation. Fixed acids entering the blood indeed generate CO_2. But they also consume bicarbonate, and just exhaling the CO_2 does not restore the bicarbonate that disappeared when the acid was added. Without actual renal excretion of those fixed acid equivalents, continuous input would soon reduce plasma bicarbonate to zero. Furthermore CO_2 cannot be converted to fixed acid and excreted in the urine. No more than a few millimoles of CO_2 are

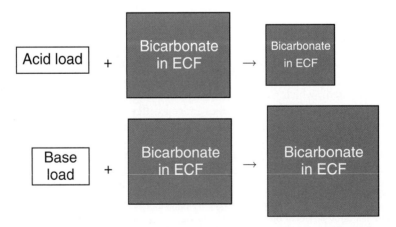

Figure 9–1. Effect of acid-base loads on bicarbonate. Acid loads combine with existing bicarbonate and reduce ECF bicarbonate. Base loads increase ECF bicarbonate.

dissolved in the daily excretion of urine, and far less carbonic acid. If somehow the kidneys could convert metabolic CO_2 to fixed acid and add it to the urine, this would generate over 10,000 milliosmoles of solute per day—clearly an impossible load to excrete.

SOURCES OF ACIDS AND BASES

Metabolism of Dietary Protein

Although the oxidative metabolism of most foodstuff is acid-base neutral, proteins contain amino acids that contribute acid or base. When sulfur-containing amino acids and those with cationic side chains are metabolized to CO_2, water, and urea, the end result is addition of fixed acid. Phosphorylated proteins also contribute to an acid load. Similarly, the oxidative metabolism of amino acids with anionic side chains adds base (consumes hydrogen ions). Depending on whether a person's diet is high in either meat or fruit and vegetables, the net input can be acid or base. For typical American diets, the input is usually acidic.

Metabolism of Dietary Weak Acids

Fruits and vegetables, particularly citrus fruit, contain many weak acids and the salts of those acids (i.e., they contain a weak acid, its conjugate base, a neutral cation such as potassium, and a very small amount of free hydrogen ions). We all know that citrus juice is acidic, with some fruit juices having a pH below 4.0. Interestingly, metabolism of these acidic substances *alkalinizes* the blood, sometimes called the *fruit juice paradox*. The complete oxidation of the protonated form of an organic acid (e.g., citric acid) to CO_2 and water is acid-base neutral, no different in principle than the oxidation of glucose. However, the complete oxidation of the base form adds bicarbonate to the body, because organic anions are precursors of bicarbonate. One can think of metabolizing an organic base anion as taking a hydrogen ion from the body fluids to protonate the anion, thus converting it to a neutral acid, and then oxidizing the acid. The loss of the hydrogen ion, as emphasized above, adds bicarbonate. This loss of hydrogen ions greatly exceeds the number of free hydrogen ions present in the original fruit juice. Although the pH of fruit juice is low, there is far more base than free hydrogen ions. Before oxidation, the mixture is acidic, but on complete oxidation to CO_2 and water, the result is addition of base.

GI Secretions

The GI tract, from the salivary glands to the colon, is lined with an epithelium and glands that secrete hydrogen ions, bicarbonate, or both. In addition, the major exocrine secretions of the pancreas and liver that flow into the duodenum contain large amounts of bicarbonate. To accomplish these tasks, the GI tract (and the kidneys as we discuss later) use the CO_2-bicarbonate system in an ingenious way. When we combine CO_2 and water to generate bicarbonate and protons within a cell, the result is always acidification of the cytosol, because the concentration of

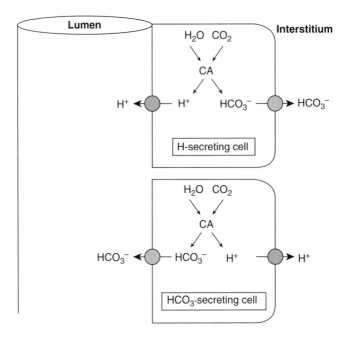

Figure 9–2. Generic model of hydrogen ion secretion (upper cell) and bicarbonate secretion (lower cell). The source of secreted ions is CO_2 and water. Every hydrogen ion moved out of a cell across one membrane must be accompanied by the transport of a bicarbonate ion out of the cell across the opposite membrane.

free protons rises. However, cells of the GI tract then *separate* the protons from the bicarbonate. They transport protons out of the cell in one direction (e.g., into the lumen of the GI tract), and bicarbonate out the other side (e.g., into the interstitium bathing the basolateral surface). Therefore the lumen becomes acidified and the surroundings (and therefore the blood leaving the tissue) becomes alkalinized (see Figure 9–2). In other regions of the GI tract, the cells reverse the direction of these processes, that is, they transport bicarbonate into the lumen (alkalinizing it) and protons into the surroundings. Thus, different regions of the GI acidify or alkalinize the blood. Normally, the sum of GI tract secretions is nearly acid-base neutral i.e. the secretion of acid at one site (e.g., the stomach) is balanced by the secretion of bicarbonate elsewhere (e.g., the pancreas). Typically, there is a small net secretion of bicarbonate into the lumen of the colon, resulting in addition of protons to the blood. However, in conditions of vomiting or diarrhea, one kind of secretion may vastly exceed the other, resulting in a major loss of acid or base from the body with a major retention of base or acid in the blood.

Anaerobic Metabolism of Carbohydrate and Fat

The normal oxidative metabolism of carbohydrate and fat is acid-base neutral. Both carbohydrate (glucose) and triglycerides are oxidized to CO_2 and water.

Although there are intermediates in the metabolism (e.g., pyruvate) that are acids or bases, the sum of all the reactions is neutral. However, some conditions lead to production of fixed acids. The anaerobic metabolism of carbohydrate produces a fixed acid (lactic acid). In conditions of poor tissue perfusion or strenuous exercise, this can be a major acidifying factor. The metabolism of triglyceride to β-hydroxybutyrate and acetoacetate also adds fixed acid (ketone bodies). These processes normally do not add much of an acid load but can add a huge acid load in unusual metabolic conditions (e.g., severe uncontrolled diabetes mellitus).

Intravenous Solutions: Lactated Ringer's

Another way in which acid-base loads can enter the body is via intravenous solutions. Hospitalized patients receive a variety of intravenous solutions; a common one being *lactated Ringer's solution*, a mixture of salts that contains lactate at a concentration of 28 mEq/L. The pH is about 6.5. However, this is an *alkalinizing* solution for the same reason described as the fruit juice paradox earlier. Lactate is an organic anion, the conjugate base of lactic acid, and when oxidized to CO_2 and water, it takes a hydrogen ion from the body fluids, thereby producing bicarbonate. Lactated Ringer's should not be confused with a *lactic acidosis* associated with certain forms of shock. In those situations the body produces equal numbers of hydrogen ions and lactate, and the result is to acidify the body fluids.

RENAL TRANSPORT OF ACIDS AND BASES

A simplified overview of the renal processing of acids and bases is as follows: The acid-base component of highest concentration in the blood is bicarbonate (24–28 mEq/L). Bicarbonate is freely filtered, and even under unusual circumstances the kidneys have to reabsorb the vast majority of the filtered load. This is accomplished primarily in the proximal tubule, thus conserving plasma bicarbonate. By itself this doesn't change things in the body; it is simply transferring the filtered bicarbonate back into the blood. The proximal tubule also secretes limited amounts of organic bases or weak organic acids and acid equivalents as previously described in Chapter 5. Then, in the distal nephron (mostly the collecting tubules), the kidneys secrete either protons or bicarbonate to balance the net input into the body (summarized in Table 9–1).

Reabsorption of Bicarbonate

The first task is always to reabsorb most of the filtered bicarbonate. Bicarbonate is freely filtered. Reabsorption is an active process via two parallel routes. The major route is an acid-base process involving the secretion of hydrogen ions. The basic principal is the same as secretion in the GI tract illustrated in the upper part of Figure 9–2. Within the tubular cells, hydrogen ions and bicarbonate are generated from CO_2 and water, catalyzed by carbonic anhydrase. The hydrogen ions are actively secreted into the tubular lumen in exchange for sodium via an antiporter (mostly) or via a primary H-ATPase.

Table 9–1. Normal contributions of tubular segments to renal hydrogen ion balance

Proximal tubule
Reabsorbs majority of filtered bicarbonate (normally about 80%)
Produces and secretes ammonium
Thick ascending limb of Henle's loop
Reabsorbs most of remaining filtered bicarbonate (normally about 10%–15%)
Distal nephron
Reabsorbs virtually all remaining filtered bicarbonate as well as any secreted bicarbonate (type A intercalated cells)
Acidifies tubular fluid (type A intercalated cells)
Secretes bicarbonate (type B intercalated cells)
Secretes ammonia and ammonium (type A and non-A, non-B intercalated cells)

Those hydrogen ions combine with *filtered* bicarbonate to form water and carbon dioxide; thus, the filtered bicarbonate "disappears." Since each of the many liters of filtrate contains bicarbonate in the range of 24 to 28 mEq/L, an enormous amount of hydrogen ion secretion occurs in the proximal tubule. At the same time, the *cellular* bicarbonate is transported across the basolateral membrane into the interstitial fluid and then into the peritubular capillary blood. The overall result from the secretion of hydrogen ions is that most of the bicarbonate filtered from the blood at the renal corpuscle is converted to CO_2 and water, and is replaced by bicarbonate generated inside the cell. It is also important to note that the hydrogen ion that was secreted into the lumen is not excreted in the urine. It has been incorporated into water.

> *Most filtered bicarbonate is recovered by combining it with secreted hydrogen ions, turning it into CO_2 and water, while simultaneously generating intracellular bicarbonate and transporting it to the interstitium.*

The secondary route for bicarbonate reabsorption is via a sodium-bicarbonate symporter that moves bicarbonate from the lumen into the cell. This bicarbonate mixes with the cellular bicarbonate and is exported across the basolateral membrane.

Specific transporters are required for these transmembrane movements of sodium, hydrogen ions, and bicarbonate. Particularly prominent in the apical membrane of the proximal tubule is the Na-H antiporter NHE3 as described in Chapter 4 and shown in Figure 9–3. This transporter is the major means not only of hydrogen ion secretion but also of sodium uptake from the proximal tubule lumen. The same NHE3 antiporter also mediates hydrogen ion secretion in the thick ascending limb. A primary H-ATPase also secretes hydrogen ions in the proximal tubule. The bicarbonate that enters in symport with sodium enters via a member

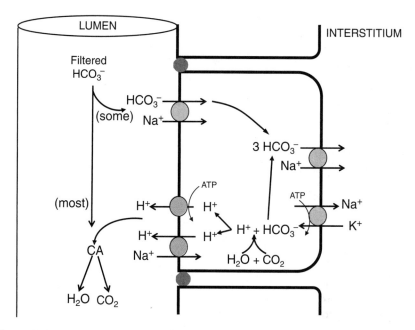

Figure 9–3. Predominant proximal tubule mechanisms for reabsorption of bicarbonate. Hydrogen ions and bicarbonate are produced intracellularly. The bicarbonate generated within the cell is transported into the interstitium via Na-3HCO$_3$ symporter (member of the NBC family). Most of the hydrogen ions are secreted via a Na-H antiporter (member of the NHE family); while some are secreted via an H-ATPase. Additional bicarbonate enters the cells via an Na-bicarbonate symporter (another member of the NBC family with 1-to-1 stoichiometry) and leaves via the Na-3HCO$_3$ symporter. The process is ultimately powered by the Na-K-ATPase that creates the sodium gradient that drives the Na-H antiporter.

of the NBC family of transporters. In the distal nephron there are segments that secrete hydrogen ions using primary active H-ATPases. The type A intercalated cells of the collecting-duct system possess this primary active H-ATPase as well as a primary active H-K-ATPase, which simultaneously moves hydrogen ions into the lumen and potassium into the cell, both actively (Figure 9–4A).

Depending on the tubular segment, the basolateral membrane exit step for bicarbonate is via a Cl-HCO$_3$ antiporter or a Na-3HCO$_3$ symporter, another member of the NBC transporter family (Figures 9–3 and 9–4A). In both cases, the movement of bicarbonate out of the cell is down its electrochemical gradient (i.e., the exit step is passive). In the proximal tubule, symport with sodium is the dominant means. Interestingly, bicarbonate both enters and exits the proximal tubular cells in symport with sodium. The key to the direction of movement is the stoichiometry of the transporter. The apical NBC transporter has a 1-to-1 ratio of bicarbonate to sodium. Since the electrochemical gradient for sodium is larger than that for bicarbonate, the movement carries both into the cell. However, the

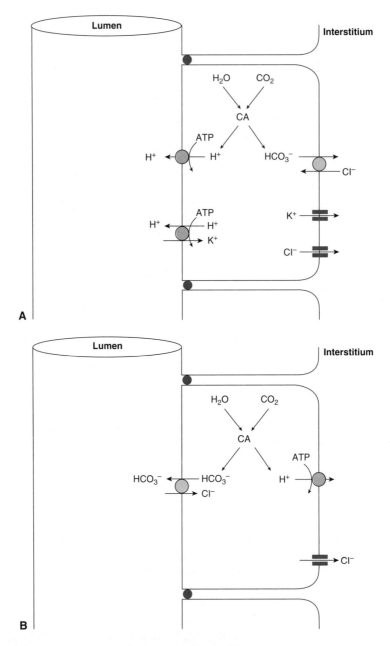

Figure 9–4. Type A and type B intercalated cells. **A,** Predominant mechanisms in type A intercalated cells for the secretion of hydrogen ions that result in formation of titratable acidity. The apical membrane contains H-ATPases and H-K-ATPases, which transport hydrogen ions alone or in exchange for potassium. Bicarbonate moves across the basolateral membrane predominantly via the AE1 antiporter. **B,** The type B intercalated cell secretes bicarbonate via the pendrin antiporter and simultaneously transports hydrogen ions into the interstitium.

basolateral NBC transporter has a 3-to-1 ratio of bicarbonate to sodium, which energetically favors export, something like a pulley system where three small weights have a greater combined weight than a single larger weight. Note that none of this can occur without the Na-K-ATPase that sets up the original sodium gradient to power the Na-H exchanger in the apical membrane.

The proximal tubule reabsorbs 80% to 90% of the filtered bicarbonate. The thick ascending limb of Henle's loop reabsorbs another 10%, and almost all the remaining bicarbonate is reabsorbed in the distal nephron (although this depends on diet and other conditions; see later discussion).

Throughout the tubule, intracellular carbonic anhydrase is involved in the reactions generating hydrogen ion and bicarbonate. In the proximal tubule, carbonic anhydrase is also located in the lumen-facing surface of apical cell membranes, and this carbonic anhydrase catalyzes the intraluminal generation of CO_2 and water from the large quantities of secreted hydrogen ions combining with filtered bicarbonate.

Acid or base loads, regardless of original source, are turned into an excess or deficit of bicarbonate.

Acid and Base Excretion

Although urine is usually acidic, it must be emphasized that neither filtration nor excretion of *free* hydrogen ions makes a significant contribution to hydrogen ion excretion. First, the filtered load of free hydrogen ions, when the plasma pH is 7.4 (40 nmolar/H^+), is less than 0.1 mmol/day. Second, there is a minimum urinary pH—approximately 4.4—that can be achieved. This corresponds to a free hydrogen ion concentration of 0.04 mmol/L. With a typical daily urine output of 1.5 L, the excretion of *free* hydrogen ions, even at the most acidic pH, could only be 0.06 mmol/day, a tiny fraction of the normal 50 to 100 mmol of hydrogen ion ingested or produced every day. To excrete these additional amounts of protons, they must associate with tubular bases.

However, acid or base loads generated from the processes described earlier result in changes in plasma bicarbonate. In essence, an acid or base load, regardless of original source, is turned into an excess or deficit of bicarbonate. The task of the kidneys is to excrete the excess or replace the deficit.[3] In response to base loads the process is relatively straightforward: The kidneys reabsorb most of the filtered bicarbonate, but excrete just enough in the urine to match the input. The kidneys do this in two ways: (1) allow *some* filtered bicarbonate to pass through to the urine and (2) secrete bicarbonate via type B intercalated cells in the distal nephron. The type B intercalated cell reverses the location of the relevant transporters found in the type A intercalated cell (Figure 9–4B). Within the cytosol, hydrogen ions and bicarbonate are generated via carbonic anhydrase. However, the H-ATPase

---

[3] Acid-base loads are partly buffered by non-bicarbonate blood buffers and intracellular buffers. Eventually, however, those buffers must release the loads they have taken up and this again turns into changes in plasma bicarbonate.

transporter is located in the basolateral membrane, and the Cl-HCO_3 antiporter, called *pendrin*, is in the apical membrane. Accordingly, bicarbonate moves into the tubular lumen via pendrin, and hydrogen ions are actively transported out of the cell across the basolateral membrane and enter the blood, where they combine with bicarbonate ions and reduce plasma bicarbonate. Thus, the overall process achieves the disappearance of excess plasma bicarbonate and the excretion of bicarbonate in the urine.

How do the kidneys excrete an *acid* load, that is, replace a bicarbonate deficit? First, be aware that generating bicarbonate from CO_2 and water simultaneously generates hydrogen ions. The hydrogen ions must be *separated* from the bicarbonate and *excreted*, otherwise these components just recombine and accomplish nothing. The process begins by reabsorbing all the filtered bicarbonate. Then, the kidneys secrete additional hydrogen ions (via H-ATPases in type A intercalated cells) that attach to bases in the tubular fluid *other than bicarbonate*. The now protonated base is excreted. Simultaneously the bicarbonate generated in the intercalated cell is transported across the basolateral membrane into the blood via Cl-HCO_3 antiporters called *AE1*, replacing the bicarbonate lost when the acid load entered the body. We emphasize again that both parts of this process must occur, that is, generation of new bicarbonate and excretion of hydrogen ions on non-bicarbonate bases. If there were no new bicarbonate, plasma levels would not be restored, and if hydrogen ions were not excreted, they would recombine with the bicarbonate just generated.

Hydrogen Ion Excretion on Urinary Bases

We see that hydrogen ion secretion can lead to both reabsorption of bicarbonate (without new bicarbonate in the proximal nephron), and acid excretion *with* addition of new bicarbonate to the blood (in the distal nephron). At first glance, this seems like a contradiction: How can the same process produce two different results? The answer lies in the fate of the hydrogen ion once it is in the lumen. For secreted hydrogen ions that combine with bicarbonate (a process that always occurs in the proximal tubule), we are simply replacing filtered bicarbonate that would otherwise have left the body. The hydrogen ion is incorporated into water. In contrast, when secreted hydrogen ions combine with a *non-bicarbonate* base in the lumen of the distal nephron, where little if any bicarbonate remains, the hydrogen ion is excreted with the base and the bicarbonate produced in the cell which is transported across the basolateral membrane into the blood is *new* bicarbonate, not a replacement for filtered bicarbonate.

Phosphate and Organic Anions

There are two sources of urinary non-bicarbonate bases: filtration and synthesis. Normally, the most important filtered base is phosphate, while ammonia is the most important synthesized base. Free plasma phosphate exists as a mixture of monovalent (acid) and divalent forms (base). As shown in

Equation 9-5, monovalent dihydrogen phosphate (on the left) is a weak acid, and divalent monohydrogen phosphate (on the right) is its conjugate base.

$$H_2PO_4^- \leftrightarrow HPO_4^{2-} + H^+ \qquad \text{Equation 9-5}$$

We can write this in the form of the Henderson-Hasselbalch equation:

$$pH = 6.8 + \log[HPO_4^{2-}]/[H_2PO_4^-] \qquad \text{Equation 9-6}$$

At the normal plasma pH of (7.4), we find that about 80% of the plasma (and filtered) phosphate is in the base (divalent) form and 20% is in the acid (monovalent) form. Much of the filtered phosphate is reabsorbed in the proximal tubule, but the rest flows on to the distal nephron. As hydrogen ions are secreted in the collecting ducts and tubular pH falls, the remaining base form takes up secreted hydrogen ions. Depending on final urine pH, the majority of the base (HPO_4^{2-}) becomes protonated to acid ($H_2PO_4^-$) and is excreted, and the bicarbonate that was simultaneously generated intracellularly enters the blood. How much phosphate is available for this process? The amount is somewhat variable, depending on a number of factors (see Chapter 10), but a typical plasma concentration is about 1 mmol/L, of which about 90% is free (the rest being loosely bound to plasma proteins). At a GFR of 180 L/day, the total filtered load of phosphate is about 160 mmol/day. The fraction reabsorbed is also variable: from 75% to 90%. Thus, unreabsorbed divalent phosphate available to take up secreted hydrogen ions amounts to roughly 40 mmol/day. In other words, the kidneys can excrete acid loads using the filtered phosphate at a rate of about 40 mmol/day. Figure 9–5 illustrates the sequence of events that achieves hydrogen ion excretion on filtered phosphate and the addition of new bicarbonate to the blood.

Acid excretion simultaneously regenerates bicarbonate.

Hydrogen Ion Excretion as Ammonium

Ordinarily, hydrogen ion excretion associated with phosphate and other filtered bases is not sufficient to balance the normal hydrogen ion production of 50 to 100 mmol/day, nor can it take care of any unusually high production of acid loads. To excrete the rest of the hydrogen ions and achieve balance, there is a second means of excreting hydrogen ions that involves ammoniagenesis and excretion of hydrogen ions as ammonium. Quantitatively, far more hydrogen ions can be excreted by means of ammonium than via filtered bases. Furthermore, while the amount of filtered base cannot be easily changed to serve the needs of acid-base balance, ammoniagenesis can be greatly increased in response to high acid loads. There are many nuances to hydrogen ion excretion via ammonium, but the basic concepts are straightforward.

 As described in Chapter 5, the catabolism of protein and oxidation of the constituent amino acids by the liver generates CO_2, water, urea, and some glutamine. Although the metabolism of the side chains of amino acids

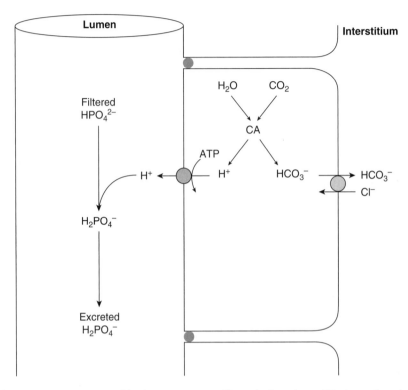

Figure 9–5. Excretion of hydrogen ions on filtered phosphate. Divalent phosphate (base form) that has been filtered and not reabsorbed reaches the collecting tubule, where it combines with secreted hydrogen ions to form monovalent phosphate (acid form), which is then excreted in the urine. The bicarbonate entering the blood is new bicarbonate, not merely a replacement for filtered bicarbonate.

can lead to addition of acid or base, the processing of the core of an amino acid—the carboxyl group and amino group—is acid-base neutral. After many intermediate steps, processing of the carboxyl group of the amino acid produces bicarbonate, and processing of the amino group produces ammonium (NH_4^+), which is the protonated form of ammonia (NH_3). Processing does not stop there, however, because ammonium in more than miniscule levels is quite toxic. Ammonium is further processed by the liver to either urea or glutamine. In both cases, each ammonium that is consumed also consumes a bicarbonate. Thus, the bicarbonate produced from the carboxyl group is just an intermediate, consumed as fast as it is made, and the process as a whole is acid-base neutral. We can write this process schematically as follows:

$$2 \text{ amino acids} \rightarrow 2NH_4^+ + 2HCO_3^- \rightarrow \text{urea or glutamine} \qquad \text{Equation 9-7}$$

When either urea or glutamine is excreted, the body has completed the catabolism of protein in a manner that promotes total body nitrogen balance, and is acid-base neutral.

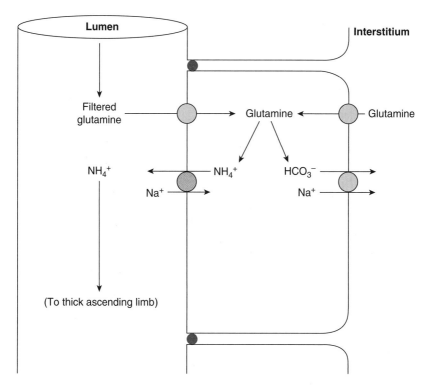

Figure 9–6. Ammoniagenesis and excretion. Ammonium production from glutamine. Glutamine is originally synthesized in the liver from NH_4^+ and bicarbonate. When glutamine reaches the proximal tubule cells, it is converted via several intermediate steps (not shown) back to NH_4^+ and bicarbonate. The bicarbonate is transported into the blood and the ammonium is secreted.

The renal handling of urea is somewhat complicated from an osmotic point of view, as described in earlier chapters, but is acid-base neutral. The renal handling of glutamine, however, is different. Although the production of glutamine by the liver is acid-base neutral, it is helpful to recognize that glutamine can be thought of as containing the two components from which it was synthesized: a base component (bicarbonate) and an acid component (ammonium). Ammonium is an acid because it contains a dissociable proton as shown in Equation 9-8. The pK of ammonium is near 9.2, making it an extremely *weak* acid (i.e., only at high pH will it release its proton), but it is an acid nevertheless. At physiological pH, over 98% of the total exists as ammonium, and less than 2% exists as ammonia. For renal acid-base purposes, this is a good thing because virtually all excreted ammonia is in the protonated form and takes a hydrogen ion with it.

$$NH_4^+ \leftrightarrow H^+ + NH_3 \qquad \text{Equation 9-8}$$

Glutamine released from the liver is taken up by proximal tubule cells, both from the lumen (filtered glutamine) and from the renal interstitium via Na-glutamine symporters. The cells of the proximal tubule then convert the glutamine back to bicarbonate and NH_4^+, in essence reversing what the liver has done. The NH_4^+ is secreted into the lumen of the proximal tubule, and the bicarbonate exits into the interstitium and then into the blood (Figure 9–6). This is *new* bicarbonate, just like the new bicarbonate generated by titrating non-bicarbonate bases. The ammonium ion has interesting chemical properties in that it can "masquerade" as other ions, in some cases as a hydrogen ion and in other cases as a potassium ion. This is because some transporters and some channels are not completely selective for the species they usually move compared to ammonium. As the concentration of ammonium rises, there is an increasing tendency for ammonium to substitute for these other ions and "sneak" its way across membranes.

Large acid loads are excreted mainly in the form of ammonium.

Also, whenever ammonium is present in body fluids, a small fraction (2% at physiological pH) always exists as ammonia, because the dissociation, although limited in extent, is nearly instantaneous. Ammonium, being a small hydrated ion, is essentially impermeant in lipid bilayers and must be handled by channels or transporters if it is to move across membranes. The neutral ammonia has low, but finite lipid bilayer permeability. More importantly, there are uniporters for ammonia, members of the Rh glycoprotein family, which transport ammonia in some regions of the nephron. In terms of cellular handling, cells sometimes transport ammonium as such and at other times transport ammonia and a proton in parallel; the end result being the same in both cases.

It would "make sense" if the ammonium secreted into the proximal tubule remained in the tubule and was excreted, but the kidneys have evolved a more complicated way of doing things. Several transporters participate in moving ammonium or ammonia into or out of the tubule in various segments. However, when ammonium produced from glutamine ends up being excreted, the process accomplishes the goal of excreting acid, regardless of intervening steps. Not all renal ammonium is excreted; some is returned to the circulation and metabolized by the liver back to urea, consuming bicarbonate in the process, thereby nullifying the renal generation of bicarbonate.

Most of the ammonium synthesized from glutamine intracellularly in the proximal tubule is secreted via the NHE3 antiporter in exchange for sodium, with ammonium substituting for a hydrogen ion (Figure 9–6). The next major transport event occurs in the thick ascending limb. In this segment about 80% of the tubular ammonium is reabsorbed, mostly by the Na-K-2Cl multiporter, with ammonium now substituting for potassium, and exits via an antiporter in exchange for sodium (Figure 9–7). In the medullary portions of the thick ascending limb this reabsorption results in accumulation of ammonium (and therefore some ammonia) in the interstitium, with the concentration progressively increasing toward the papilla, analogous to the osmotic gradient. Finally, in the medullary collecting ducts there is secretion once again. Ammonia is taken up from the interstitium primarily via Rh glycoprotein uniporters, with some ammonium taken up via the Na-K-ATPase (with ammonium substituting for potassium). Ammonia exits into the lumen via an apical Rh glycoprotein and combines with a hydrogen ion secreted via an

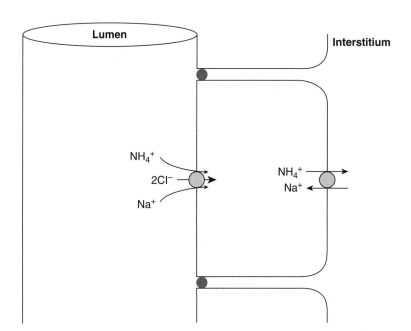

Figure 9–7. Ammonium reabsorption in the thick ascending limb. Ammonium reaches the thick ascending limb from two sources. Most comes as a result of secretion in the proximal tubule. Some also enters the thin limbs from the medullary interstitium in the form of neutral ammonia and is subsequently reprotonated in the lumen (ammonium recycling). Ammonium is reabsorbed in the thick ascending limb by several mechanisms, the predominant one being entrance via the NKCC multiporter (where ammonium substitutes for potassium) and exit via a sodium-ammonium antiporter (NHE-4).

H-ATPase (Figure 9–8). Thus, the ammonium that was reabsorbed in the thick ascending limb and accumulated in the medullary interstitium is now put back into the tubule and excreted. The processes of excreting acid and base are summarized in Figure 9–9.

Quantification of Renal Acid-Base Excretion

We can quantify the excretion of acid-base equivalents by looking at three quantities in the urine: (1) the amount of *titratable acidity*, (2) the amount of ammonium, and (3) the amount of bicarbonate, if any. Titratable acidity represents the amount of acid that was taken up by urinary bases other than ammonia. It can be measured by titrating the urine with strong base (NaOH) to a pH of 7.4. (The amount of NaOH required to increase the pH back to 7.4 thus equals the amount of hydrogen ion that was secreted and combined with phosphate and organic bases.) Urinary ammonium equals the urinary volume times the urinary ammonium concentration. (Ammonium does not contribute to titratable acidity because with a pK of 9.2, few hydrogen ions are removed by titration to pH 7.4.) Similarly, urinary bicarbonate equals the urinary volume times the urinary bicarbonate concentration.

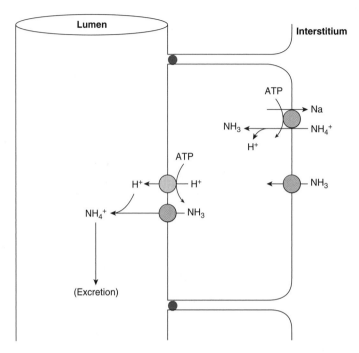

Figure 9–8. Ammonium secretion in the inner medulla. Several mechanisms are involved. A prominent one involves uptake and secretion of neutral ammonia via specific transporters in parallel with hydrogen ion secretion, resulting in reformation of ammonium in the lumen. In the innermost medulla, the high interstitial ammonium concentration allows ammonium to substitute for potassium on the Na-K-ATPase.

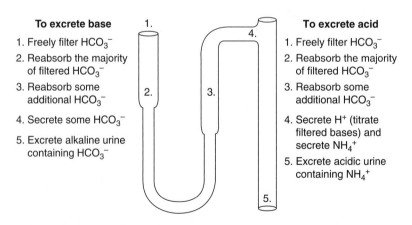

To excrete base

1. Freely filter HCO_3^-
2. Reabsorb the majority of filtered HCO_3^-
3. Reabsorb some additional HCO_3^-
4. Secrete some HCO_3^-
5. Excrete alkaline urine containing HCO_3^-

To excrete acid

1. Freely filter HCO_3^-
2. Reabsorb the majority of filtered HCO_3^-
3. Reabsorb some additional HCO_3^-
4. Secrete H^+ (titrate filtered bases) and secrete NH_4^+
5. Excrete acidic urine containing NH_4^+

Figure 9–9. Overall scheme for excretion of acid and base. In all cases the majority of filtered bicarbonate is reabsorbed. For base excretion, some filtered bicarbonate moves through to be excreted along with some additional bicarbonate secreted by type B intercalated cells in the distal nephron. For acid excretion all the filtered bicarbonate is reabsorbed. Then hydrogen ions are secreted in the distal nephron, contributing to titratable acidity. Ammonium excretion accounts for the bulk of acid excretion.

Table 9–2. Renal contribution of new bicarbonate to the blood in different states

	Alkalosis	Normal state	Acidosis
Titratable acid (mmol/day)	0	20	40
Plus NH_4^+ excreted (mmol/day)	0	40	160
Minus HCO_3^- excreted (mmol/day)	80	1	0
Total added to body (mmol/day)	–80	59	200
Urine pH	8.0	6.0	4.6

Thus, we can write the net acid excretion as:

$$\text{Net acid excretion} = \text{titratable acid excreted} + NH_4^+ \text{ excreted} - HCO_3^- \text{ excreted}$$
$$\text{Equation 9-9}$$

Note that there is no term for free hydrogen ion in the urine because, even at a minimum urine pH of 4.4, the number of free hydrogen ions is trivial.

Typical urine data for the amounts of bicarbonate contributed to the blood by the kidneys in three potential acid-base states are given in Table 9–2. Note that in response to acidosis, as emphasized previously, increased production and excretion of NH_4^+ is quantitatively much more important than increased formation of titratable acid.

REGULATION OF THE RENAL HANDLING OF ACIDS AND BASES

The kidneys respond to acute acid-base loads by moving transporters for hydrogen ions and bicarbonate (H-ATPases and Cl-HCO₃ antiporters) back and forth between intracellular vesicles and surface membranes. Acid loads increase the number of H-ATPases in the apical membrane of type A intercalated cells, while also increasing Cl-HCO₃ antiporters (AE1) in the basolateral membrane. Analogously, base loads shift Cl-HCO₃ antiporters (pendrin) into the apical membrane of type B intercalated cells and H-ATPases into the basolateral membrane. Chronic acid-base loads lead to gradual shifts in transporter expression on a slower time scale and an actual interconversion between some type A and type B intercalated cells. There is also a shift in the production of glutamine and abundance of ammonia transporters. All of these processes change the relative amount of hydrogen ion and bicarbonate secretion. While some hormones, specifically aldosterone, alter renal acid-base transporter activity, these hormones are generally regulated by the body for purposes other than acid-base balance. Aldosterone probably plays more of a permissive role (*allows* transporter function) than a controlling role.

There are no known neural or hormonal signals that specifically convey acid-base information to the kidneys, leaving us with the question: how do the kidneys detect the acid-base status of the body? The answer seems to lie in a constellation of responsive elements within the kidneys themselves that detect extracellular pH, intracellular pH, and intracellular bicarbonate. There are pH-dependent membrane receptors that activate G-protein-coupled signaling pathways and there are pH-dependent ion channels. These proteins serve as extracellular pH detectors. There are also a multitude of intracellular enzymes whose activity varies with pH and/or bicarbonate concentration. The combination of pH and bicarbonate detection serves as de facto PCO_2 detection. In effect, the kidneys act as "pH meters," bicarbonate detectors, and PCO_2 detectors and adjust their transport of hydrogen ion and bicarbonate excretion accordingly.

Control of Renal Glutamine Metabolism and Ammonium Excretion

In addition to regulating hydrogen ion and bicarbonate secretion per se, there are several homeostatic controls over the production and tubular handling of NH_4^+. First, the generation of glutamine by the liver is increased by low plasma pH. In this case, the liver shifts some of the disposal of ammonium ion from urea to glutamine. Second, the renal metabolism of glutamine is also subject to control by extracellular pH. A decrease in extracellular pH stimulates renal glutamine uptake and oxidation by the proximal tubule, whereas an increase does just the opposite. Thus, an acidosis that lowers plasma pH, by stimulating renal glutamine oxidation, causes the kidneys to contribute more new bicarbonate to the blood, thereby counteracting the acidosis. This pH responsiveness increases over the first few days of an acidosis and allows the glutamine-NH_4^+ mechanism for new bicarbonate generation to become the predominant renal process for opposing the acidosis. Conversely, an alkalosis inhibits glutamine metabolism, resulting in little or no renal contribution of new bicarbonate via this route.

Table 9–3 provides a summary of the processes of adding acids and bases to the body fluids. The unifying and, therefore, simplifying principle is that all processes of acid or base addition boil down to addition or loss of bicarbonate. All processes

Table 9–3. Summary of processes that acidify or alkalinize the blood

Non-renal mechanisms that acidify the blood
Consumption and metabolism of protein (meat) containing acidic or sulfur-containing amino acids
Consumption of acidic drugs
Metabolism of substrate without complete oxidation (fat to ketones and carbohydrate to lactic acid)
GI tract secretion of bicarbonate (puts acid in blood)

Non-renal mechanisms that alkalinize the blood
Consumption and metabolism of fruit and vegetables containing basic amino acids or the salts of weak acids
Consumption of antacids
Infusion of lactated Ringer's solution
GI tract secretion of acid (puts bicarbonate in the blood)

Renal mechanisms that acidify the blood
Allow some filtered bicarbonate to pass into the urine
Secrete bicarbonate

Renal means that alkalinize the blood
Secrete protons that form urine titratable acidity
Excrete NH_4^+ synthesized from glutamine

that acidify the blood remove bicarbonate, and all processes that alkalinize the blood add bicarbonate.

ACID-BASE DISORDERS AND THEIR COMPENSATION

In this section we briefly address the topic of acid-base disorders in the context of the kidney. While many acid-base disorders involve complex pathology, they manifest themselves as deviations in levels of either arterial PCO_2, bicarbonate, or both. Clinicians assign acid-base disorders to four categories: (1) high pCO_2 is a *respiratory acidosis*, (2) low pCO_2 is a *respiratory alkalosis*, (3) low bicarbonate is a *metabolic acidosis*, and (4) high bicarbonate is a *metabolic alkalosis*.[4] Respiratory disorders are caused by over- or under-ventilation relative to the rate of metabolism while metabolic disorders have many causes.

$$pH = 6.1 + \log[\text{bicarbonate}]/0.03\ PCO_2 \qquad \text{Equation 9-10}$$

It should be clear from the Henderson-Hasselbalch equation for the CO_2-bicarbonate buffer system (Equation 9-10) that changing either the PCO_2 or changing the bicarbonate concentration raises or lowers the pH. If only one of these is changed, it is called a *primary uncompensated disorder*. In most cases the situation is more complicated because there is at least some, and usually considerable *compensation*. Compensation arises when either PCO_2 or bicarbonate levels remain altered for a period of time and the body changes the other variable in the *same direction*. By doing so, the *ratio* of bicarbonate to PCO_2 is brought closer to normal, and therefore the pH is closer to normal. For example, if the PCO_2 is abnormally low, renal compensation consists of reducing plasma bicarbonate. The compensatory change brings the ratio of bicarbonate to PCO_2 closer to a normal value, and therefore the pH is closer to normal. However, compensation for an acid-base disorder is not *correction*, because even if the compensation has returned the pH to the normal range, both PCO_2 and bicarbonate values are still abnormal. Consider a case where the PCO_2 is too high (respiratory acidosis) due to hypoventilation. The body compensates by increasing bicarbonate. If bicarbonate is increased high enough, this restores pH to the normal range; however, it doesn't correct the original respiratory problem that resulted in an elevated PCO_2. The same logic applies to any other acid-base disorder.

The astute reader may recognize a potential problem in the interpretation of acid-base disorders. When any acid-base disorder is *well compensated*, that is, the degree of compensation is such that the pH is in the normal range, both the PCO_2 and bicarbonate are elevated or depressed in the same direction. How do we know which variable is the primary disturbance and which is altered due to compensation? Suppose both the PCO_2 and bicarbonate are high. Is this respiratory acidosis with renal compensation, or is it metabolic alkalosis with respiratory

---

[4] Strictly speaking, altered plasma pH is an "*emia*" meaning in the blood, as in acidemia and alkalemia, while an "*osis*" is a *process* that adds acid or base to the blood. For example, a metabolic alkalosis adds bicarbonate to the blood and creates an alkalemia. Most sources blur the distinction between these terms.

compensation? Fortunately in a clinical setting it would be rare not to have additional information. For example, the high PCO_2 of an emphysema patient is, in all likelihood, a respiratory acidosis resulting from impaired ventilation, not a compensation for a metabolic alkalosis. Nevertheless, in real life there are often mixed acid-base disorders that indeed present a diagnostic challenge in the clinic.

Renal Response to Respiratory Acidosis and Alkalosis

In a respiratory acidosis, low alveolar ventilation that might be caused, for example, by chronic obstructive pulmonary disease (COPD) causes an increase in PCO_2, in turn causing a decrease in pH. The pH could be restored to normal if the bicarbonate were increased to the same degree as PCO_2. The healthy kidneys respond to the increased PCO_2 by contributing new bicarbonate to the blood in the manner previously described.

The renal compensation in response to respiratory alkalosis is just the opposite. Respiratory alkalosis is the result of hyperventilation, as occurs at high altitude, in which the person transiently eliminates carbon dioxide faster than it is produced, thereby lowering PCO_2 and raising pH. The decreased PCO_2 and increase in extracellular pH signal reduced tubular hydrogen ion secretion and increased bicarbonate secretion. Bicarbonate is lost from the body and the loss results in decreased plasma bicarbonate and a return of plasma pH toward normal. There is no titratable acid in the urine (the urine is alkaline in these conditions), and there is little NH_4^+ in the urine because the alkalosis inhibits NH_4^+ production and excretion.

Renal Response to Metabolic Acidosis

There are many possible causes of metabolic acidosis, including the kidneys themselves (see below) due either to increased input of acid (by ingestion, infusion, or production) or direct loss of bicarbonate from the GI tract, as in diarrhea. Whether there is loss of bicarbonate or addition of hydrogen ions, the result is the same: a depressed level of bicarbonate and low plasma pH. The renal response (if the kidneys are not the cause) is to produce more bicarbonate, thereby returning pH toward normal. (Note that this is a response, not compensation, because the primary problem is not a respiratory change in PCO_2.) To do this, the kidneys must reabsorb all the filtered bicarbonate and contribute new bicarbonate through increased formation and excretion of NH_4^+ and titratable acid. This is precisely what normal kidneys do in the case of any acid load. If the acid load is too great or the problem originates in the kidneys themselves, the bicarbonate concentration will remain low.

> Compensation helps normalize
> pH but does not correct the
> original disturbance.

Renal Tubular Acidosis (RTA)

We see that the kidneys respond to a metabolic acidosis by increasing acid excretion, simultaneously generating bicarbonate to replace that being consumed by the acidosis. There is also a group of disorders in which the kidneys themselves create the acidosis, either due to renal transport defects or abnormal signaling to the kidneys. This group is called *renal tubular acidosis* (RTA). These disorders are classified (with an admittedly confusing numbering system) as proximal RTA (type 2), classical distal RTA (type 1), hyperkalemic RTA (type 4), and finally type 3, which is rare and represents a combination of types 1 and 2.

Proximal RTA is a defect in the bicarbonate reabsorbing capacity in the proximal tubule. It allows large amounts of bicarbonate to flow on to the distal nephron. Proximal RTA usually occurs as a component of generalized proximal tubule transport failure called *Fanconi's syndrome* in which the transport of almost all substances in the proximal tubule is impaired, leading, for example, to excretion of organic substances that are normally completely reabsorbed. Hydrogen ion secretion (and bicarbonate generation) is normal in the distal nephron, but the large load of bicarbonate that would normally have been reabsorbed upstream overwhelms the transport capacity of the distal nephron and bicarbonate is excreted. Plasma bicarbonate then falls until the filtered load is reduced enough to match the finite but limited reabsorptive capacity of the nephron. The urine is acidic due to distal hydrogen ion secretion, and plasma bicarbonate stabilizes at a low value (typically ~15 mEq/L). Proximal RTA is often accompanied by hypokalemia. This occurs because the large load of unreabsorbed solute reaching the distal nephron stimulates potassium secretion in a manner similar to the action of loop and thiazide diuretics (see Chapter 8).

Classical *distal RTA* (called type 1 because it was the first to be identified) is a defect in acid secretion by type A intercalated cells in the distal nephron. These cells are responsible for acidifying the urine following normal bicarbonate reabsorption and are therefore responsible for net acid excretion. In distal RTA they fail to do this, due either to defects in the basolateral H-Cl antiporter AE1 or the apical H-ATPase. As a result the kidneys have difficulty excreting normal net acid loads via titration of filtered bases, but can excrete enough ammonium to maintain balance. As with proximal RTA, type 1 RTA is often accompanied by hypokalemia.[5]

Hyperkalemic RTA (type 4) is a component of the renal transport defects associated with hypoaldosteronism (low secretion of aldosterone) or pseudohypoaldosteronism (failure to respond to aldosterone). As described in Chapter 8, these defects decrease potassium secretion and create hyperkalemia. Simultaneously the hyperkalemia reduces both the ability to take up glutamine and synthesize ammonium in the proximal tubule and transport it into the medullary collecting duct. The result is that ammonium excretion cannot be increased enough to take care of acid loads and metabolic acidosis ensues.

---

[5] While failure of the basolateral H-Cl antiporter would block operation of both the apical H-ATPase and the apical H-K-ATPase that reabsorb potassium, there is presently no agreed upon mechanistic explanation for the hypokalemia.

KEY CONCEPTS

 ① Plasma pH is regulated by controlling the concentrations of CO_2 (PCO_2) and bicarbonate.

 ② Fixed acid or base loads are metabolized into excesses or deficits of bicarbonate in the body.

 ③ Fixed acids and bases can enter the body via GI processes, metabolism, intravenous infusions, and renal processes.

 ④ Under all conditions, the kidneys must recover virtually all filtered bicarbonate.

 ⑤ The kidneys excrete acid by attaching secreted hydrogen ions to filtered or synthesized urinary bases.

 ⑥ Phosphate is the most important filtered urinary base.

 ⑦ A large fraction of an acid load is excreted by converting glutamine to bicarbonate and ammonium, then excreting the ammonium and returning the bicarbonate to the blood.

 ⑧ Primary acid-base disorders that alter either PCO_2 or bicarbonate can be compensated by changing the other variable in the same direction, thereby preserving the ratio of bicarbonate to PCO_2.

 ⑨ Several forms of renal tubular acidosis (RTA) result from inability to secrete enough hydrogen ions to match normal input.

 STUDY QUESTIONS

9–1. A patient excretes 2 L of urine at a pH of 7.4. The urine bicarbonate concentration is 5 mEq/L. What is the titratable acid excretion?

    a. It is 10 mEq.

    b. It is negative 10 mEq.

    c. It is zero.

    d. Cannot determine without data for ammonium.

9–2. Which of the following is an acid load per se or becomes an acid load after metabolism?

a. Eating a large steak.

b. Eating unsweetened grapefruit juice.

c. Eating sweetened grapefruit juice.

d. Intravenous infusion of sodium lactate.

9–3. How does the proximal tubule handle the majority of the filtered bicarbonate?

a. Bicarbonate diffuses into tubular cells on a uniporter.

b. Bicarbonate is taken up by the tubular cells via antiport with small base anions (e.g., formate).

c. Bicarbonate is taken up by the tubular the cells via antiport with chloride.

d. Bicarbonate combines with a proton in the lumen and is converted to carbon dioxide and water.

9–4. In which situation(s) would you expect to see decreased or no renal excretion of acid equivalents?

a. During a major metabolic acidosis such as diabetic ketoacidosis.

b. During a time when the pancreas is secreting a high amount of bicarbonate-rich fluid into the GI tract.

c. In response to consuming a large number of antacid tablets.

d. All of these situations.

9–5. What is the fate of ammonium secreted in the proximal tubule?

a. It flows through to the urine.

b. It is mostly reabsorbed in the collecting ducts.

c. It is mostly reabsorbed in the thick ascending limb and secreted again in the collecting ducts.

d. It is mostly reabsorbed in the thick ascending limb and combined with bicarbonate to form urea.

9–6. A person develops a decreased arterial PCO_2 because of hyperventilation. If this condition persists, what response would we expect by the kidneys?

a. More urinary titratable acidity.

b. More urinary bicarbonate.

c. More urinary ammonium.

d. A decreased urinary pH.

Regulation of Calcium, Magnesium, and Phosphate

10

OBJECTIVES

- ▶ State the normal total plasma calcium concentration and the fraction that is free.
- ▶ Describe the distribution of calcium between bone and extracellular fluid and the role of bone in regulating extracellular calcium.
- ▶ Describe and compare the roles of the gastrointestinal tract and kidneys in calcium balance.
- ▶ Describe and compare bone remodeling and plasma calcium buffering by bone.
- ▶ Describe the role of vitamin D in calcium balance.
- ▶ Describe how the synthesis of the active form of vitamin D (calcitriol) is regulated.
- ▶ Describe the regulation of parathyroid hormone secretion and state the major actions of parathyroid hormone.
- ▶ Describe the renal handling of phosphate.
- ▶ Describe how parathyroid hormone changes renal phosphate excretion.
- ▶ Describe the control of FGF23 production and its actions in the kidney.
- ▶ Describe the major features of magnesium balance.

OVERVIEW

Calcium, magnesium, and phosphorus (in the form of phosphate) are major elemental constituents of the body, the majority of all of them being components of bone. Most of the non-bone fractions are compartmentalized in organelles within cells or complexed with cytosolic proteins, and only small fractions of any of these substances are free in the ECF. However, plasma levels of the free form of these ions, even though representing small percentages of total body amounts, are crucial for body function. Deviations lead to serious, even life-threatening pathologies. Calcium and phosphate are usually discussed together because both their physiological roles and mechanisms of regulation are intertwined. All three substances are regulated by cooperative interactions between the kidneys, the GI tract, and bone.

The Chemistry of Calcium, Magnesium, and Phosphate

The physiology and regulation of calcium, magnesium, and phosphate are critically dependent on their chemical properties. Calcium and magnesium are both divalent alkali metal cations that play similar roles in some contexts and different roles in others. Their free (non-complexed) concentrations in the ECF are roughly the same (~1 mM), low enough so that they are not significant components of plasma osmolality. However, being divalent, they are major contributors to the layer of cations that are attracted to negative charges on plasma membranes and large plasma proteins. Alterations in plasma levels of either one of these species have major effects on the behavior of excitable cells because they alter the electric field sensed by voltage-gated channels. In contrast, their intracellular levels are vastly different from each other and these ions perform very different functions. Most intracellular magnesium is complexed with ATP or other negatively charged molecules. The concentration of the free dissolved component is about 0.5 mM, only slightly lower than in the ECF. In contrast, the free intracellular calcium concentration is less than 1000th of magnesium. This difference and their different functional roles within cells are due to nuances of their chemistry.

As with all inorganic ions, calcium and magnesium are surrounded by hydration shells of water. Calcium is a larger ion and holds its water less tightly, while the smaller magnesium holds water more tightly. Thus magnesium, with its more strongly held water, actually has a larger effective volume in solution. This permits magnesium to enter magnesium-selective channels that accommodate the hydrated ion, but excludes magnesium from reaching restricted binding sites in proteins that are accessible to dehydrated calcium. A number of intracellular proteins possess binding sites for calcium and serve as calcium detectors. This allows very small changes in free intracellular calcium to be effective modulators of protein function in the face of a large background concentration of magnesium. Free intracellular calcium rises in brief bursts as components of intracellular signaling cascades, perhaps like a small flashlight intermittently illuminating parts of a dark room, while magnesium is like a floodlight of constant brightness.

Phosphate is the substance we previously encountered in Chapter 9 in association with titratable acidity. In the plasma it exists primarily as a mix of monovalent ($H_2PO_4^-$) and divalent phosphate (HPO_4^{2-}), with a summed concentration of about 1 mM. A significant property of phosphate is its tendency to combine with calcium in various stoichiometric ratios and form insoluble complexes. In bone this tendency to precipitate is crucial for the formation and maintenance of bone structure, but when it occurs elsewhere in the body it leads to soft tissue calcification. This chemical property is a major reason why plasma phosphate levels must be controlled. Within the renal tubules calcium may combine with phosphate or oxalate and form renal calculi (kidney stones) that can grow large enough to block the ureter.

The Physiology of Calcium

Calcium plays several roles in the body. First, it is a major constituent of bone, which contains 99% of total-body calcium. Second, it is used in cells as a second messenger, allowing for rapid transmission of signals from surface membrane channels or receptors to promote various cellular actions. Third, its presence in the ECF stabilizes the electrical sensitivity of voltage-gated membrane channels. Normal total plasma calcium is about 10 mg/dL (2.5 mM), of which about 1 mM is in the free ionized form. Another 1 mM of the total is reversibly bound to plasma proteins such as albumin, and the rest is complexed to anions with relatively low molecular weights, such as citrate and phosphate.

All body cells regulate free cytosolic calcium concentrations to very low levels in order to prevent formation of calcium complexes with the many forms of phosphate within cells, and to prevent inappropriate activation of signaling pathways. They do this with a variety of active transport systems (ATPases and antiporters) that remove calcium from the cytosol, either to the external medium or to intracellular organelles.

Calcium in the ECF is the source for calcium entering cells through calcium channels and is the calcium that triggers rapid exocytosis of neurotransmitters and signals contraction in smooth and cardiac muscle cells. As indicated earlier, the diffuse layer of extracellular cations associated with negatively charged membranes affects voltage-gated channels. Low levels of calcium fool sodium channels into sensing more depolarization than actually exists, leading to spontaneous firing of motor neurons. In turn, this firing triggers inappropriate muscle contraction, called *low-calcium tetany*. If severe enough, it leads to respiratory arrest because of spasms in the ventilatory muscles.[1]

An important modulator of the effect of calcium on nerve membranes is the plasma pH. Serum albumin has many anionic sites that reversibly bind both protons and calcium. These ions compete for occupancy of the binding sites. As pH rises, protons dissociate and calcium ions take their place, thereby lowering the concentration of free calcium ions. In turn, this reduces the diffuse cationic layer associated with cell membranes. Thus, a patient with an acute alkalosis is more susceptible to tetany, whereas someone with acidosis will not manifest tetany at levels of total plasma calcium low enough to cause symptoms in normal people.

> Plasma calcium is tightly regulated by moving calcium in and out of bone.

Elevated plasma calcium (hypercalcemia) is also a serious medical problem, particularly if the rise occurs rapidly. Hypercalcemia has multiple effects, again resulting from an effect on excitable cell function. Hypercalcemia leads to CNS depression, muscle weakness, and GI tract immotility.

---

[1] Even though calcium in the extracellular medium is required to trigger the release of neurotransmitter from motor neurons (absence of calcium blocks this process completely), low calcium causes excessive muscle stimulation because hyperexcitability is manifested at calcium levels well above the extremely low levels needed to block exocytosis.

② Moment-to-moment regulation of plasma calcium is achieved, not by input and output from the body, but rather by moving calcium in and out of bone. The majority of bone substance consists of *hydroxyapatite*, a complex of calcium, phosphate, and hydroxyl groups.[2] Bone stores of calcium are an enormous buffer system that keeps plasma calcium nearly constant regardless of whole body balance. Thus, ordinary variations in ingestion and excretion of calcium have little effect on plasma levels because of this tight buffering. The long-term regulation of total calcium in bone is, of course, important for bone growth during childhood and bone integrity in adult life. Here the kidneys play an important but indirect role because (1) they excrete calcium in the urine and (2) are involved in forming the active form of vitamin D, which is a major controller of gastrointestinal calcium absorption.

EFFECTOR SITES FOR CALCIUM BALANCE

GI Tract

Most dietary calcium simply passes through the GI tract to the feces. The amount absorbed depends on many factors, particularly the quantity of calcium in the diet. Some of the calcium that is absorbed moves by a regulated active transcellular process in the duodenum. The majority is absorbed by paracellular diffusion in the lower small intestine, where intestinal content spends a far greater time than the few minutes in the much shorter duodenum, and thus has greater opportunity for passive absorption. The active transport system in the duodenum plays its most important role when dietary calcium is limited. Calcium enters duodenal cells passively through calcium-selective channels (members of the TRP family), binds reversibly to mobile cytosolic calcium-binding proteins (called *calbindins*), and is then actively transported out the basolateral side via a Ca-ATPase and to some extent by a Na-Ca antiporter. Calbindins contain multiple binding sites for calcium and are free to diffuse throughout the cytosol. They act as delivery trucks for calcium, permitting large amounts of calcium to move from place to place within a cell, in this case from apical to basolateral membrane, all the while keeping the concentration of *free* calcium at a low level (see Figure 10–1).

> *The GI tract absorbs less than half of dietary calcium.*

Kidneys

③ The kidneys handle calcium by filtration and reabsorption. There is no secretion. Overall reabsorption of the filtered load is normally 98%, leaving only 2% to be excreted. The free component of plasma calcium (about 40%) is freely filterable. About 65% of the filtered load is reabsorbed in the

---

[2]Apatites are a class of compounds of variable structural formula that usually include calcium, phosphate, and an anion such as fluoride, chloride, or hydroxide. The apatites in bone are a mixture of these, but the dominant one is hydroxyapatite.

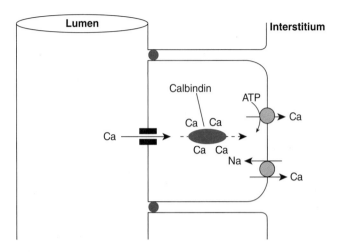

Figure 10–1. Generic method for transcellular calcium transport in the GI tract and kidney. In all body cells the free intracellular calcium concentration must be kept to minuscule levels to prevent formation of insoluble complexes and activation of deleterious signaling pathways, even though the concentrations of calcium at the two external surfaces of the cells are thousands of times higher. The epithelial cells accomplish this by using diffusible calbindins. As calcium enters the cells through channels in the luminal surface this slightly raises the calcium concentration in the microenvironment near the channels, thus promoting the binding of calcium to calbindins. At the basolateral surface active extrusion of calcium via ATPases and sodium-calcium antiporters lowers the calcium concentration in the local microenvironment, promoting dissociation of calcium from the calbindins.

proximal tubule. Another 20% is reabsorbed in the thick ascending limb of Henle's loop, and almost all the rest in the distal convoluted tubule and connecting tubule.

Calcium reabsorption in the proximal tubule and thick ascending limb of Henle's loop is passive and paracellular. Whereas the tight junctions in many regions of the tubule are impermeable to cations, the tight junctions in the proximal tubule and thick ascending limb permit passive cation flux. Water reabsorption in the proximal tubule concentrates tubular calcium and drives paracellular flux, while the lumen-positive potential in the thick ascending limb is the major driving force. In both cases the driving forces are dependent directly or indirectly on active sodium reabsorption as they are for so many other substances. In the distal tubule calcium reabsorption is active and transcellular. It uses the same general mechanism as in the GI tract, that is, entrance via calcium-specific TRP channels, diffusion bound to calbindins and active exit across the basolateral membrane by a combination of Ca-ATPase and Na-Ca antiport activity (Figure 10–2). Endocrine control of renal calcium handling is exerted in the distal tubule.

The amount of calcium excreted in the urine, when averaged over time, is equal to the net addition of new calcium to the body from the GI tract (recall that most dietary calcium is excreted directly and is not absorbed). Thus, the kidneys participate in maintaining a stable balance of total-body calcium. The change in renal excretion in response to changes in dietary input is much slower than the

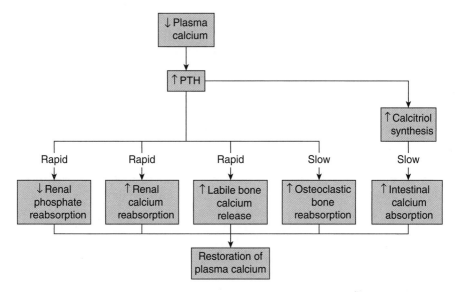

Figure 10–2. Responses to reduced plasma calcium concentration. Reduced plasma calcium stimulates secretion of PTH. Bone immediately releases calcium from the labile pool into the ECF both stimulated by PTH and independently. PTH also stimulates renal calcium reabsorption and reduces phosphate reabsorption, thereby lowering plasma phosphate and preventing formation of calcium phosphate complexes. On a slower time scale PTH stimulates osteoclastic bone resorption and increased synthesis of calcitriol from vitamin D in the kidney, leading to increased calcium absorption from the GI tract.

equivalent responses to dietary sodium, water, or potassium. For example, only about 5% of an increment in dietary calcium appears in the urine, whereas virtually all of an increased ingestion of water soon appears in the urine. The reason is that most of the dietary increment never gains entry to the blood because it fails to be absorbed from the GI tract. In contrast, when dietary intake of calcium is reduced to extremely low levels, there is a gradual reduction of urinary calcium.

What determines renal calcium excretion? While the filtered load is somewhat variable, being the product of free plasma calcium and GFR, the GFR is stabilized by processes not related to calcium. In fact, an increase in urinary calcium excretion can be induced simply by administering saline. This feature is used clinically as an emergency procedure when calcium levels in the blood get alarmingly high, the treatment consisting of administering large amounts of saline, with the consequence that large amounts of calcium-containing fluid pass through the kidneys to the urine. Independent, calcium-specific regulation of calcium excretion is exerted in the distal tubule via control of active calcium reabsorption. We will describe this control shortly.

Bone

Bone is a complex tissue structurally and physiologically. It is the least understood, but in some ways the most important of the major effector systems for calcium management. Bone contains 99% of total-body calcium, primarily in the form of hydroxyapatite that is deposited on a tough collagen network. The equilibrium between crystalline hydroxyapatite and its dissolved components is highly labile, dependent on the local concentrations of calcium, phosphate, hydrogen ions, and specific non-collagenous proteins in the immediate environment. Bone is penetrated by a labyrinth of tiny passageways containing fluid (bone fluid), cells (mostly osteocytes), and, in the larger passageways, blood vessels. Osteocytes deep within bone communicate with each other and surface cells via long cellular extensions containing gap junctions. Calcium moves back and forth between the bone surface and the inner recesses via this cellular network.

Bone fluid is separated from the ECF by a layer of surface-lining cells. These cells are flattened versions of the active osteoblasts involved in forming bone and bone remodeling (see below). The flux of calcium through or around the surface-lining cells is crucial in regulating the concentration of calcium in the ECF. Details of how this occurs are unclear, but the result is clear: flux of calcium from a labile pool within bone is a powerful short-term buffering system that prevents large swings in plasma calcium concentration. It does not require hormonal signals. However, the set point for plasma calcium concentration maintained by the rapid movement of calcium in and out of bone is critically regulated by hormonal control, as discussed later.

There is a second flux process between bone and plasma involving calcium called bone *remodeling* that affects calcium stores on a slower time scale. Remodeling, while it includes calcium, is directed toward maintaining the mechanical properties of bone rather than calcium levels in the blood. Remodeling consists of the simultaneous actions of giant, multinucleated cells called *osteoclasts* that erode little pits in the bone matrix, and their partners, nearby *osteoblasts*, which follow behind and fill in the pits with new bone matrix (like brick masons replacing bricks in a wall one brick at a time). The osteoclasts pump hydrogen ions and create an acidic micro space directly underneath them that solubilizes hydroxyapatite. The calcium and phosphate freed up by this process is then transported transcellularly by the osteoclasts to the ECF. The daily flux of calcium via remodeling is much less than that associated with rapid flux associated with the normal buffering by bone of plasma calcium described above. Normally the fluxes associated with remodeling result in no net gain or loss of calcium, but imbalance in resorption of bone matrix relative to replacement causes gradual loss of bone density and pathology such as osteoporosis.

THE PHYSIOLOGY OF PHOSPHATE

About 85% of total-body phosphate is located in bone as a partner with calcium in hydroxyapatite. Another 14% of body phosphate is located intracellularly in the form of a multitude of phosphorylated proteins and metabolic intermediates. The remaining 1% is in the ECF. Phosphate is plentiful in the diet, as it is contained in all proteins. The fraction absorbed from the GI tract varies somewhat with circumstances, typically being about 65% of the ingested amount, so that the total amount absorbed varies more or less directly with dietary input. Accordingly, regulation of body phosphate is exerted mainly via excretion by the kidneys. Phosphate absorption from the GI tract occurs throughout the small intestine by paracellular diffusion and by transcellular active transport. The active component uses several different Na-phosphate symporters in the apical membrane to bring phosphate into the intestinal enterocytes. The exit step is not characterized, but is presumed to be via a phosphate uniporter.

In the blood, approximately 5% to 10% of the phosphate is protein bound, so that 90% to 95% is filterable at the renal corpuscle. Normally, approximately 75% of this filtered phosphate is actively reabsorbed in the proximal tubule. The mechanism uses the same Na-phosphate symporters as in the GI tract.

As with other substances handled by filtration and tubular reabsorption, the rate of phosphate excretion can be changed by altering the filtered load or the rate of reabsorption. Even relatively small increases in plasma phosphate concentration (and, hence, filtered load) can produce relatively large increases in phosphate excretion. This occurs when plasma phosphate concentration increases as a result of increased dietary phosphate intake or release of phosphate from bone. The Na-phosphate symporters are a tubular maximum-limited (T_m) system, and the normal filtered load is just a little higher than the T_m. This means that most of the filtered phosphate is reabsorbed, but some spills into the urine. It also means that the reabsorptive capacity is saturated in normal conditions, and any increase in filtered load simply adds to the amount excreted.

HORMONAL CONTROL OF CALCIUM AND PHOSPHATE

Calcium and phosphate are regulated by a web of interacting signals. For this reason, we describe the regulation of both substances together. Control systems have two purposes: (1) on a short-term basis to keep the plasma level of calcium within a range that does not perturb excitable cell function and (2) on a longer term basis to ensure that there is enough total calcium and phosphate in the body to maintain bone integrity. The key hormones that directly control calcium and phosphate are the active form of vitamin D (1,25-$(OH)_2$D), parathyroid hormone (PTH), and fibroblast growth factor 23 (FGF23).[3] These hormones regulate three crucial processes: (1) the input of calcium and phosphate into the body from the GI tract, (2) the excretion of calcium and phosphate by the kidneys, and (3) the movement of both substances between plasma and bone. These hormones also regulate the production of each other.

Vitamin D

The term vitamin D in common use denotes any member of a family of closely related molecules that are derived from cholesterol. One member, called vitamin D_3 (cholecalciferol), is synthesized in the skin by the action of ultraviolet radiation on precursors synthesized in the body. Another member, vitamin D_2 (ergocalciferol),

---

[3] Another hormone—calcitonin, also called thyrocalcitonin because it is produced by parafollicular cells in the thyroid gland, affects plasma calcium by reducing osteoclastic bone resorption. However, it has minimal effectiveness in humans and is not necessary for normal calcium homeostasis. A synthetic, more potent form is sometimes employed as a pharmacological agent to treat osteoporosis.

is ingested in food derived from plants. Vitamin D supplements may contain either one. Although not identical structurally, vitamins D_2 and D_3 are equivalent in terms of their physiological roles in the body and can be considered to be the same vitamin. Ingested vitamin D has no significant biological activity by itself. It must be hydroxylated at the 1 and 25 positions to be active. Ingested vitamin D travels in the blood and becomes hydroxylated at the 25 position by the liver and then hydroxylated again at the 1 position by proximal tubular cells within the kidneys to yield the active form, which is now, strictly speaking, a hormone. When the precursor is cholecalciferol (vitamin D_3), the active hormone is also called calcitriol. For the rest of this text, we will use calcitriol to denote the active hormone that is recognized by specific receptors in target tissues.

The hydroxylation step occurring in the kidneys that produces calcitriol is the key control point in its production. That step is regulated by PTH and FGF23. Specifically, PTH stimulates this step (produces more calcitriol), while FGF23 inhibits it.

The major action of calcitriol on effector systems is to stimulate transcellular absorption of calcium, and to a lesser extent, phosphate, by the duodenum. It also increases passive calcium absorption in the lower small intestine by effects on tight junctions. As well, it stimulates the renal-tubular reabsorption of both calcium and phosphate. Its primary mode of action is to increase the genetic expression of the protein components in the transport pathways. These actions serve functionally to increase or preserve the supply of the main building blocks for the synthesis of hydroxyapatite in bone, that is, calcitriol is effectively a bone-promoting hormone. Calcitriol also has some complicated actions on bone cells best characterized as permissive for normal bone turnover. The influences of calcitriol on bone and the kidney are far less important than its actions on the GI tract to stimulate absorption of calcium (and phosphate).

In terms of the other hormones, calcitriol inhibits the synthesis of PTH in the parathyroid glands. Since PTH stimulates calcitriol production, this action completes a classic negative feedback loop that maintains normal levels of both hormones. Calcitriol also stimulates production of FGF23.

The major event in calcitriol deficiency is decreased calcium absorption from the GI tract, resulting in decreased availability of calcium for bone formation or reformation. In children, the newly formed bone protein matrix fails to be calcified normally because of the low availability of calcium, leading to the disease Rickets.[4]

PTH

The parathyroid glands are small (pea sized or less) nodules of tissue embedded within the thyroid gland in the neck. Normally a person has four parathyroid glands. They secrete PTH (parathyroid hormone), an 84-amino peptide hormone. The GI tract, kidneys, and bone are all subject to direct or indirect control by

---

[4]Rickets, osteomalacia, and osteoporosis are characterized by low calcium content in bone. Rickets and osteomalacia are commonly associated with a low *supply* of calcium, typically because of low vitamin D. Osteoporosis seems to represent improper *regulation*, so that the ongoing bone-forming and bone-dissolving processes are dominated by bone dissolution.

PTH. All of its normal activity is contained in the first 34 amino acids, and synthetic PTH can be made containing only this component. The PTH half-life in the plasma is very short (<10 minutes), mostly due to rapid degradation in the liver,[5] with renal filtration and uptake playing a secondary role. PTH secretion is controlled on a moment-to-moment basis by the calcium concentration of the ECF bathing the cells of the parathyroid glands. *Decreased* plasma calcium concentration stimulates PTH secretion, and increased plasma concentration inhibits secretion. Extracellular calcium acts directly on the parathyroid glands by binding to a novel class of calcium receptors coupled to G-protein-linked signaling cascades that inhibit the secretion of PTH. Low extracellular calcium stimulates PTH secretion by removing a tonic inhibition. This is a sensitive control system designed to keep free plasma calcium at about 1 mM.

> *Vitamin D controls the **supply** of calcium; PTH controls calcium concentration.*

Another regulator is plasma phosphate. Elevated phosphate *stimulates* PTH secretion by stimulating the capacity of the parathyroid gland to synthesize PTH, so that chronically high levels of phosphate lead to elevated PTH. A third regulator, as mentioned previously, is calcitriol, which inhibits PTH synthesis. On a moment-to-moment basis, calcium is the primary *acute* regulator.

PTH exerts at least five distinct effects on calcium and phosphate homeostasis (summarized in Figure 10–2 showing the response to hypocalcemia).

1. PTH actions on bone acutely increase the movement of calcium and phosphate from the labile pool in bone into the ECF. The mechanism of action is not clear, but the effect is to raise the set point for plasma calcium between plasma and bone fluid, that is, net efflux continues until plasma calcium rises to a new level.

2. PTH stimulates the bone remodeling process. Normal remodeling results in no net change in total bone calcium, but when PTH remains elevated the result is erosion of bone hydroxyapatite.

3. PTH stimulates the hydroxylation step in the kidneys that generates calcitriol. The increased calcitriol stimulates calcium uptake from the GI tract and ensures that enough new calcium enters the body to replace losses in the urine.

4. PTH increases renal tubular calcium reabsorption, mainly by an action on the distal convoluted tubule. At this location it acts rapidly through activation of kinases that phosphorylate regulatory proteins on a short-term basis. It also acts, on a slower time scale, to increase synthesis of all the components of the transport pathway. The increased uptake of calcium from the tubular lumen increases basolateral extrusion (by a combination of Ca-ATPase activity and Na-Ca antiporter activity). The overall effect is to decrease urinary calcium excretion and retain body calcium.

---

[5] In breaking down PTH, the liver releases peptide fragments that are active hormones in their own right, but with actions different from PTH. These fragments act to oppose the normal actions of PTH.

5.   PTH *reduces* the proximal tubular reabsorption of phosphate, thereby increasing urinary phosphate excretion and decreasing extracellular phosphate concentration.

The adaptive value of the first four effects in the above list all result in a higher extracellular calcium concentration and thus compensate for the lower calcium concentration that originally stimulated PTH secretion. When PTH acts on bone, both calcium and phosphate are released into the blood. Similarly, calcitriol enhances the intestinal absorption of both calcium and phosphate, so that the processes that restore calcium to its normal level are simultaneously acting to increase the plasma phosphate *above* normal.

> *PTH increases plasma calcium and **decreases** plasma phosphate.*

But this is an unwanted action because of the tendency to form insoluble precipitates of calcium phosphate. Under the influence of PTH, plasma phosphate does not actually increase, because of PTH's *inhibition* of tubular phosphate reabsorption. Indeed, this effect is so potent that plasma phosphate may actually decrease when PTH levels are elevated.

There are nuances to the actions of PTH on bone that have important clinical implications. The response of bone to PTH depends on the pattern of its plasma concentration over time. PTH can either promote resorption of hydroxyapatite (its usual action) or, if administered intermittently, promote deposition. Primary hyperparathyroidism, resulting from a primary defect in the parathyroid glands (e.g., a hormone-secreting tumor), generates a continuous excess hormone level and causes enhanced bone resorption. This leads to bone thinning and the formation of completely calcium-free areas or cysts. In this condition plasma calcium often increases and plasma phosphate decreases; the latter caused by increased urinary phosphate excretion. A seeming paradox is that urinary calcium excretion is *increased* despite the fact that tubular calcium reabsorption is enhanced by PTH. The reason is that the elevated plasma calcium concentration induced by the effects of PTH causes the filtered load of calcium to increase even more than it increases the reabsorptive rate. Because the filtered load is so great, there is also an increased amount *not* reabsorbed (i.e., excreted). This result nicely illustrates the necessity of taking both filtration and reabsorption (and secretion, if relevant) into account when analyzing excretory changes of any substance. And as mentioned earlier, the high urinary calcium content promotes the formation of stones.

In contrast to what happens with the continuous presence of elevated PTH that accelerates bone resorption and release of calcium, *intermittent* rises (produced by infusions once per day) actually *increase* deposition of calcium in bone. Intermittent infusion of PTH is used therapeutically to increase bone density in osteoporosis patients.

FGF23

Fibroblast growth factor 23 (FGF23) is a peptide hormone synthesized by osteoblasts and osteocytes in bone. It is primarily a negative regulator of phosphate, but has indirect actions on calcium. FGF23 secretion is increased in response to elevated levels of phosphate. It is also stimulated by calcitriol. In the kidney, FGF23 receptors are located in both the proximal and distal tubules. Tubule cells contain the membrane protein *Klotho*, which is a co-receptor required in order for target cells to bind FGF23. FGF23 has two actions in the proximal tubule: (1) it decreases reabsorption of phosphate by reducing the expression of Na-phosphate symporters (an action similar to that of PTH) and (2) it decreases production of calcitriol (an action opposite to that of PTH). It does this by reducing expression of the 1-alpha hydroxylase that produces calcitriol. In the distal tubule FGF23 increases expression of the TRP channels that are the entry step for regulated calcium reabsorption.

SUMMARY OF NORMAL CALCIUM AND PHOSPHATE REGULATION

The interplay between calcitriol, PTH, and FGF23 acts to maintain adequate amounts of calcium and phosphate in bone and a normal level of free plasma calcium. Calcitriol stimulates uptake and retention of calcium and phosphate. PTH responds to changes in plasma calcium acutely to normalize plasma calcium via retrieval from a labile bone pool and by raising phosphate excretion, thereby preventing a rise in the product of calcium and phosphate concentrations that would otherwise promote soft tissue calcification. PHT also ensures an ongoing level of calcitriol and normal bone turnover via remodeling. FGF23 acts as brake on calcitriol production, preventing too much calcium and phosphate uptake, and stimulates phosphate excretion, thereby decreasing the tendency of phosphate to stimulate PTH production. Figure 10–3 shows the hormonal response to a rise in plasma phosphate, while Table 10–1 summarizes the effects of the various hormones.

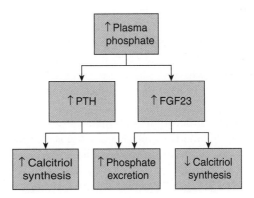

Figure 10–3. Response to rise in plasma phosphate concentration. Increased release of PTH from the parathyroid gland and FGF23 from bone both reduce phosphate reabsorption in the kidney, causing increased phosphate excretion. The two hormones exert offsetting influences on the production of calcitriol in the kidneys.

Table 10–1. Functions of major hormones that control calcium and phosphate

Hormone	Effect on Ca and phosphate	Effect on other hormones
Calcitriol	Stimulates Ca and phosphate uptake from GI tract.	Suppresses PTH synthesis.
	Stimulates renal reabsorption of Ca and phosphate. Maintains normal bone remodeling.	Stimulates FGF23 secretion.
PTH	Stimulates rapid transfer of Ca and phosphate from bone and stimulates slower bone resorption.	Stimulates renal production of calcitriol.
	Increases renal excretion of phosphate. Stimulates renal reabsorption of Ca.	
FGF23	Increases renal excretion of phosphate. Increases renal reabsorption of Ca.	Decreases renal production of calcitriol.

Chronic Renal Failure

Much of the physiology we have described is illustrated by the case of *chronic renal failure,* in which loss of functioning nephrons decreases many renal functions, including glomerular filtration rate, production of calcitriol, and excretion of phosphate. The pathophysiology demonstrates the workings of the feedback system involved in calcium and phosphate homeostasis. Decreased excretion of phosphate due to low GFR causes increased plasma phosphate (hyperphosphatemia) that in turn causes elevated levels of PTH and FGF23. High FGF23 and decrease in functioning nephrons both serve to reduce the renal production of calcitriol. The low calcitriol leads to additional problems, namely reduced calcium uptake from the GI tract and removal of the inhibitory action of calcitriol on PTH synthesis. The high PTH (secondary hyperparathyroidism) stimulates excessive bone resorption, leading to osteoporosis. Another serious complication is calcification of vascular smooth muscle, in part due to the high levels of phosphate. One goal in the treatment of hyperphosphatemia associated with chronic renal failure is reduction of phosphate absorption from the GI tract. This is accomplished by feeding the patient high doses of phosphate binders, of which calcium is one. The calcium forms complexes with phosphate in the GI tract, reducing the availability of absorbable phosphate. Another clinical intervention is to provide exogenous calcitriol. This hormone suppresses expression of the PTH gene in the parathyroid gland. It also increases GI absorption of phosphate, the very thing we are trying to inhibit, but its ability to lower the synthesis of PTH is the more important action because this reduces the excessive resorption of bone stimulated by PTH.

MAGNESIUM PHYSIOLOGY AND RENAL HANDLING

The majority of total-body magnesium exists in bone. Magnesium is not chemically linked with other components of hydroxyapatite, but is adsorbed to its surface. Most of the remaining body magnesium is located within cells where it forms complexes with ATP and serves as a cofactor for many enzymes. While the intracellular levels and functions of magnesium and calcium are quite different, their extracellular concentrations, functions, and transport are remarkably similar. As with calcium, the normal fraction of dietary magnesium absorbed from the GI tract is less than 50%. Details are lacking, but it is believed that the major absorptive mechanism is paracellular diffusion throughout the small intestine. About 60% of plasma magnesium is free, 30% is adsorbed to albumin, and the rest is complexed with small anions. The free component is freely filtered, and then handled by the nephron almost identically to calcium. About 20% of the filtered load is reabsorbed in the proximal tubule and 70% in the thick ascending limb of the loop of Henle, in both cases by the paracellular route. These are somewhat different proportions than for calcium (65% is reabsorbed in the proximal tubule) and may reflect differences in the selectivity of the tight junctions. The distal tubule actively reabsorbs magnesium. The apical influx is via a magnesium-specific class of TRP channels. This flux is driven primarily by the negative membrane potential because the free cytosolic magnesium concentration is similar to that in the lumen. The basolateral exit step is active, but its mechanism is not established. In the healthy body renal excretion of magnesium is regulated to maintain balance with input and to keep plasma levels steady. It is believed that regulation is exerted on the activity of apical membrane TRP channels, but the hormonal or other signaling pathways remain unknown.

KEY CONCEPTS

1 Calcium has a strong tendency to associate with small anions and restricted sites on proteins that are not accessible to magnesium.

2 Moment-to-moment maintenance of plasma calcium primarily involves calcium flux between bone and plasma.

3 The kidneys reabsorb almost all filtered calcium, the key site of regulation being in the distal tubule.

4 The key action of vitamin D is to ensure adequate absorption of calcium from the GI tract.

5 Regulation of calcium and phosphate are interdependent and involve interactions between calcitriol, PTH, and FGF23.

6 Keeping phosphate levels in the normal range is required to permit normal calcium deposition and retrieval from bone.

7 Magnesium is transported by the GI tract and kidney in a manner very similar to calcium.

STUDY QUESTIONS

10–1. The most important action of calcitriol is to stimulate:
   a. calcium deposition in bone.
   b. calcium resorption from bone.
   c. calcium absorption from the GI tract.
   d. calcium reabsorption from the renal tubules.

10–2. Which of the following leads to decreased levels of phosphate in the body?
   a. Adding large amounts of calcium to the diet.
   b. The actions of FGF23.
   c. The actions of PTH.
   d. All of these lead to decreased phosphate in the body.

10–3. In response to a sudden decrease in plasma calcium, what is the source for most of the calcium that restores plasma levels?
   a. Bone
   b. The GI tract
   c. The renal tubules
   d. The organelles of tissue cells

10–4. Magnesium
   a. is reabsorbed from the renal tubules primarily by paracellular diffusion.
   b. has a free cytosolic concentration far higher than that of calcium.
   c. exists in the body primarily in bone.
   d. All of the above statements are true.

10–5. In a case of acute hypercalcemia, one can rapidly lower plasma calcium and increase urinary calcium excretion by
   a. feeding large amounts of phosphate.
   b. giving large amounts of saline.
   c. injecting PTH.
   d. withholding phosphate from the diet.

10–6. Which condition(s) would directly or indirectly increase the urinary excretion of phosphate?
   a. The actions of PTH on bone.
   b. The actions of osteoclasts in bone.
   c. The actions of PTH on the kidneys.
   d. All of these would increase urinary phosphate excretion.

Answers to Study Questions

CHAPTER 1

1–1. (b)   Renal corpuscles are distributed throughout the cortex, which includes the region just above the cortico-medullary border (i.e., the juxtamedullary region). None are in the medulla.

1–2. (c)   Each glomerulus is associated with a nephron, which includes a loop of Henle. Each collecting duct is formed from the coalescence of several nephrons.

1–3. (d)   Balance implies that input equals output, which can occur at normal or abnormal levels of amounts in the body, or normal or abnormal input, so long as the inputs are matched by equal outputs.

1–4. (c)   The macula densa cells are located in the tubule where it passes between the afferent and efferent arterioles. This location is at the end of the thick ascending limb of the loop of Henle just before it becomes the distal tubule.

1–5. (d)   A healthy young 70-kg person contains about 42 L of water (~60% of body weight), and filters up to 180 L of plasma each day.

1–6. (a)   Secretion implies transport from tubular cell to the lumen. Most often the substance entered the cell from the blood, but it could also be synthesized and then transported.

CHAPTER 2

2–1. (d)   Most efferent arterioles feed peritubular capillaries, but those associated with juxtamedullary glomeruli feed vascular bundles that descend into the medulla.

2–2. (d)   While various factors affect *how much* plasma is filtered, the glycocalyx, basement membrane, and particularly the slit diaphragms bridging the foot processes of podocytes, all of which are extracellular, are the key determinants of *what* is filtered.

2–3. (a)   Rapid control is exerted over the contractile properties of vascular smooth muscle that in turn affects hydrostatic pressure in glomerular capillaries.

2–4. (d)   Other than larger molecules that are only partially or slightly filtered, the plasma concentrations of a small freely filtered substance are not altered by filtration because water and the substance in question are filtered in the same proportions.

2–5. (c) The lowering of pressure upstream from the glomerulus is offset by contraction of the efferent arteriole, an action that by itself raises glomerular capillary pressure. The net effect leaves glomerular capillary pressure almost unchanged.

2–6. (a) Glomerular capillary pressure starts at about 60 mm Hg and falls very little along the length of the capillaries. This value is far higher than in most peripheral capillaries.

CHAPTER 3

3–1. (d) The excretion rate of a substance divided by its plasma concentration yields the clearance.

3–2. (a) The metabolic clearance rate represents the sum of all clearance routes. Since there are two major routes of clearance (kidneys and feces) the metabolic clearance must be higher than either one alone. The fact that the drug has a higher urinary concentration than plasma concentration mainly reflects the reabsorption of water.

3–3. (c) In the second test both the plasma concentration and filtered load (and hence rate of excretion) are increased, yielding offsetting effects on the calculation.

3–4. (b) Normally the relative clearance rates are: PAH > creatinine ≈ inulin > urea > sodium.

3–5. (d) Anything that increases the removal of a substance from the blood, whether by increased filtration, increased metabolism, or less reabsorption, increases clearance.

CHAPTER 4

4–1. (c) 100 mmol is the amount of solute in one-third of a kilogram of filtrate (333 mL), so this much water accompanies the reabsorbed solute.

4–2. (d) Sodium enters the cells across the apical membrane by several pathways, the major one being the NHE3 antiporter.

4–3. (b) Tight junctions exhibit selectivity just as membrane transporters do. The proximal tubule tight junctions are leaky to sodium and a number of other solutes, but not glucose.

4–4. (d) In the proximal tubule water is reabsorbed both transcellularly and paracellularly.

4–5. (a) A substance moving by a T_m-limited system cannot move paracellularly. It moves transcellularly via transporters that have an upper limit to their capacity to transport.

4–6. (b) By definition multiporters move two or more different solute species simultaneously, either in the same direction (symporters) or the opposite direction (antiporters).

CHAPTER 5

5–1. (c)   The large filtered load presents more glucose than the reabsorptive T_m-limited transporters can handle. Under all conditions there is always far more filtered sodium than glucose and sodium is never rate-limiting.

5–2. (d)   Small useful organic solutes are freely filtered. They are reabsorbed transcellularly by a T_m system. The normal filtered load is below the T_m.

5–3. (a)   Anions that are secreted must enter the cell against a negative membrane potential, and usually against a concentration gradient as well; thus, they are actively transported.

5–4. (c)   Drugs that are weak bases are usually neutral (unprotonated) at high pH. This favors their passive reabsorption by simple diffusion, and therefore low excretion.

5–5. (a)   Urea becomes concentrated above plasma levels in the proximal tubule by the loss of water, and further concentrated in the descending thin limb by secretion. It is therefore quite concentrated at the hairpin turn. Its concentration reaches its highest value in the inner medullary collecting duct where little water remains.

5–6. (b)   Urea is secreted in the deep descending thin limbs where the interstitial concentration is high.

CHAPTER 6

6–1. (b)   Reabsorbed sodium must be balanced by reabsorbed anions. Once most of the bicarbonate is reabsorbed, only chloride exists in high enough concentration to match the continued reabsorption of sodium.

6–2. (b)   So long as there is filtration there is excretion of organic waste which obligates water to be excreted also.

6–3. (d)   Osmotic conditions in all tubule regions favor water reabsorption.

6–4. (a)   The tubular fluid entering the medulla is iso-osmotic. If the tubules did not separate salt from water, the medullary interstitium would remain iso-osmotic. The luminal fluid would also remain iso-osmotic because there would be no osmotic gradient to either dilute it or concentrate it.

6–5. (b)   After drinking a large amount of water there would be a decline in ADH, which would decrease water permeability in the ADH-sensitive regions of the tubule.

6–6. (b)   Under all conditions the majority of filtered water (approximately two-thirds) is reabsorbed in the proximal tubule.

CHAPTER 7

7–1. (d)   Intrarenal baroreceptors are modified smooth muscle cells in the afferent arteriole.

7–2. (a)   The action of renin to produce angiotensin I is the rate-limiting step because (1) there is excess substrate (angiotensinogen) and (2) almost all angiotensin I is converted to angiotensin II by angiotensin-converting enzyme (ACE).

7–3. (a) Consumption of salt without water concentrates the ECF and triggers secretion of ADH. A key action of ADH is to cause insertion of aquaporins into the luminal membrane of cortical collecting duct principal cells.

7–4. (c) Loss of blood volume and likely ensuing drop of arterial pressure both reduce the inhibition of sympathetic outflow (i.e., sympathetic outflow increases). A prime target of sympathetic outflow in the kidneys is the juxtaglomerular cells.

7–5. (a) Signals from the macula densa act in a paracrine manner (travel by diffusion to nearby cells) to regulate afferent arteriole smooth muscle, and thus GFR.

7–6. (b) The blocking of agents that stimulate sodium reabsorption leads to increased sodium excretion. Since dopamine is a natriuretic agent (increases sodium excretion), blocking it will *decrease* sodium excretion.

CHAPTER 8

8–1. (d) The distal nephron both reabsorbs and secretes potassium. Quantitatively the main control is exerted over the rate of secretion.

8–2. (d) The uptake of potassium from the lumen is an active process via the Na-K-2Cl multiporter, energetically driven by the sodium gradient.

8–3. (b) Even under conditions of major natriuresis, most of the filtered sodium and chloride is reabsorbed, but with a high potassium load, high secretion in the distal nephron can lead to more potassium excretion than filtration.

8–4. (b) A large dietary load of potassium is absorbed from the GI tract and taken up by tissue cells (mostly muscle), stimulated by insulin, before being released slowly and excreted.

8–5. (d) BK potassium channels in the distal nephron are activated during excretion of large potassium loads.

8–6. (a) Angiotensin II reduces potassium secretion by principal cells.

CHAPTER 9

9–1. (c) The urine is already neutral; thus, it contains no acidity that can be titrated.

9–2. (a) Animal protein, when metabolized, adds acid to the body. The other substances, when metabolized, generate bicarbonate and thus become an alkali load.

9–3. (d) Filtered bicarbonate combines with protons to become carbon dioxide and water. Simultaneously it is generated within the tubular cells and exported with sodium across the basolateral membrane.

9–4. (c) Antacid tablets constitute an alkali load that reduces or even exceeds metabolic acid production.

9–5. (c)   Ammonium is secreted in the proximal tubule, reabsorbed in the thick ascending limb, and secreted again in the medullary collecting ducts.

9–6. (b)   In response to a respiratory alkalosis the kidneys generate a compensating metabolic acidosis. Thus excrete less acid and more bicarbonate.

CHAPTER 10

10–1. (c)   Calcitriol has several actions, but the most important one is to ensure adequate supply of calcium from the GI tract.

10–2. (d)   Excess calcium in the GI tract reduces phosphate absorption, while FGF23 and PTH increase renal excretion.

10–3. (a)   There is a labile pool of calcium in bone that buffers short-term changes in plasma calcium.

10–4. (d)   Most magnesium exists in bone (although in a different state than bone calcium). Its tubular reabsorption is paracellular in the proximal tubule and thick ascending limb, and its cytosolic concentration is far higher than that of calcium.

10–5. (b)   A large saline load causes more tubular fluid to be delivered to the distal nephron; thus, higher than normal amounts of calcium-containing fluid are excreted.

10–6. (d)   PTH stimulates retrieval of both calcium and phosphate from bone, as does the action of osteoclasts. PTH decreases renal reabsorption of phosphate; thus all of these lead to increased phosphate excretion.

Appendix A

Table A–1. Summary of major reabsorption and secretion events by major tubular segments

	Proximal tubule	Loop of Henle	Distal tubule	Collecting ducts
Organic nutrients	R			
Urea	R	S		R
Proteins, peptides	R			
Phosphate	R			
Sulfate	R			
Organic anions*	S			
Organic cations*	S			
Urate	R (mostly) and S			
Sodium	R	R	R	R
Chloride	R	R	R	R
Potassium	R	R		S (usually) and R
Water	R	R		R
Hydrogen ions	S	S		S or R
Bicarbonate	R	R		S or R
Ammonium	S	R		S
Calcium	R	R	R	

*Some passive transport may occur in the distal nephron depending on pH.

Table A–2. Major functions of the various collecting-duct cells

Principal cells
1. Reabsorb sodium
2. Secrete potassium
3. Reabsorb water

Type A intercalated cells
1. Secrete hydrogen ions
2. Reabsorb or secrete potassium

Type B intercalated cells
1. Secrete bicarbonate

Inner medullary cells
1. Reabsorb urea
2. Secrete ammonia/ammonium

Appendix B

Table B–1. Classes of diuretics

Class	Mechanism	Major site affected
Carbonic anhydrase inhibitors	Inhibit secretion of hydrogen ions, which reduces reabsorption of bicarbonate and sodium	Proximal tubule
Loop diuretics	Inhibit Na-K-2Cl symporter in luminal membrane	Thick ascending limb of Henle loop
Thiazides	Inhibit Na-Cl symporter in luminal membrane	Distal convoluted tubule
Potassium-sparing diuretics	Inhibit action of aldosterone Block sodium channels	Cortical collecting tubule Cortical collecting tubule

Index

Page numbers followed by *f*, *t*, and *n* indicate figures, tables, and footnotes, respectively.